Perfectly Planned

Our best weekly plans ever!

Contents

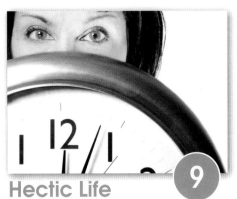
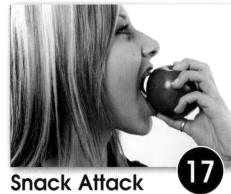
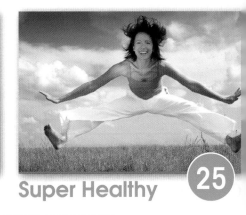
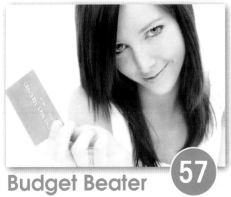
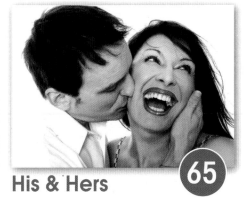
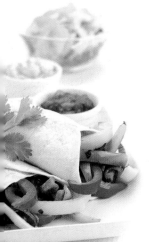

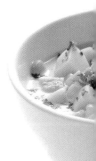

our **best weekly plans** ever!

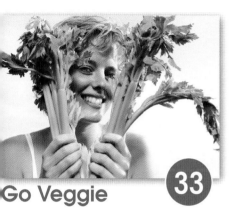 Go Veggie **33**

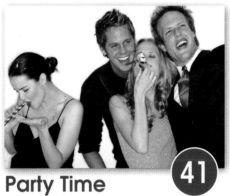 Party Time **41**

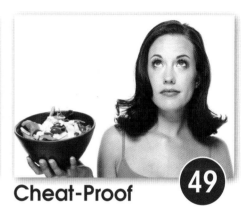 Cheat-Proof **49**

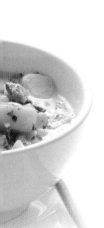 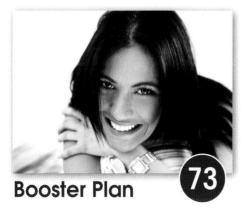 Booster Plan **73**

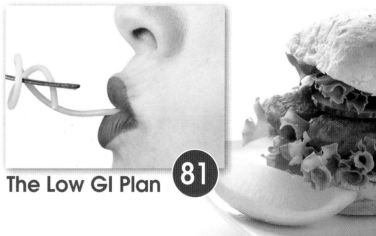 The Low GI Plan **81**

At Scottish Slimmers we believe that you are much more likely to succeed at weight loss if your eating plan can be tailored to suit you, rather than the other way around!

In this book we demonstrate just how versatile Positive Eating is with weekly plans to cover almost any lifestyle – whether you are a person looking for quick and simple meals, a student on a tight budget, keen to put health foremost, or love to party, you're sure to find something that fits the bill.

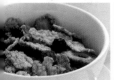
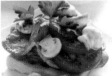
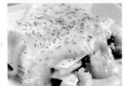
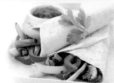
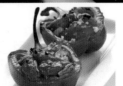
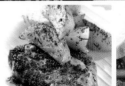

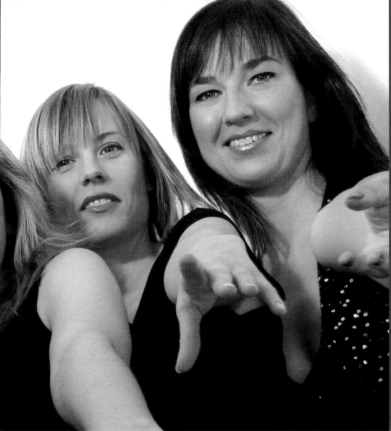
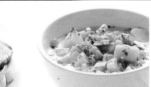
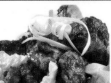

How to use
the plans...

- Do read the instructions at the beginning of each plan, so you know whether or not Every Day Bonus foods and Essential Extras have already been included, or whether you should add these yourself. A brief summary of Every Day Bonus foods follows to remind you of the choices you have.

- Although each plan is based on one week's eating, you can use them as examples to plan similar weeks of your own. As always, if there is a meal or Essential Extra you don't like, you can choose a similar alternative from your copy of the PEPplus.

- Note that any milk, yoghurt, fromage frais, cheese or fruit included in meals has not been taken from Every Day Bonus allowances and has been taken into account in the Check values given.

- Also, note how many Checks per day a plan is based on – if you are allowed more, you can add Essential Extras of your choice.

- We've done all the thinking for you, so all that's left is to choose which plan you wish to follow, check your storecupboard, write out your shopping list – and look forward to a week of successful weight loss!

Every Day Bonus Foods

Most of the plans in this book include Every Day Bonus foods, but for those where they need to be added, here is a brief reminder of what you can choose. Full details can be found in your personal copy of the PEPplus.

Remember that Every Day Bonus Foods never have to be counted from your daily Checks allowance!

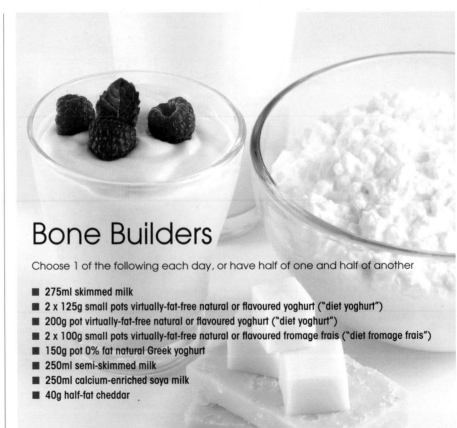

Bone Builders

Choose 1 of the following each day, or have half of one and half of another

- 275ml skimmed milk
- 2 x 125g small pots virtually-fat-free natural or flavoured yoghurt ("diet yoghurt")
- 200g pot virtually-fat-free natural or flavoured yoghurt ("diet yoghurt")
- 2 x 100g small pots virtually-fat-free natural or flavoured fromage frais ("diet fromage frais")
- 150g pot 0% fat natural Greek yoghurt
- 250ml semi-skimmed milk
- 250ml calcium-enriched soya milk
- 40g half-fat cheddar

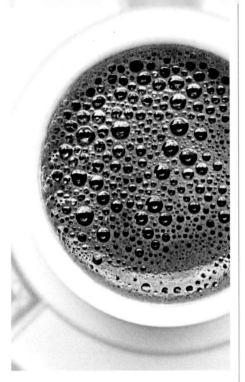

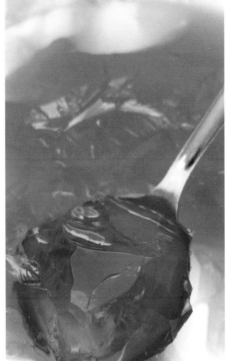

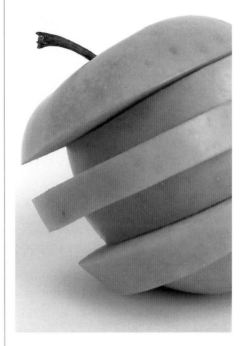

Liquid Assets

Drink 6/8 cups/glasses of fluid each day. Water, tea, coffee and diet drinks may be drunk freely.

Taste & flavour

Items such as sweeteners, herbs, spices, pepper, vinegar, lemon juice, mustard, stock cubes, yeast extract, soy sauce, Worcestershire sauce, oil-free dressings, essences, rhubarb, sugar-free jelly, sugar-free gum, and small amounts of spray oil may be used freely. Always use the minimum amount of salt.

5-a-day

Each day you should have 2 "average" servings of fruit and at least 3 servings of No-Check vegetables to reach your 5-a-day. You may have more vegetables if you wish.

Fruit

An average serving of fruit is typically one of the following:

- 1 medium round fruit such as an apple or orange or peach or nectarine or pear.
- 2 small fruits such as satsumas, figs, small kiwi fruits
- 85g grapes, 100g tropical fruits such as kumquats, lychees, physallis, 200g peeled melon, 225g berries
- 100g canned fruit in juice, 100ml unsweetened fruit juice

Two average servings are typically one of the following:
1 large cooking apple, 1 medium banana, 1 medium mango or papaya

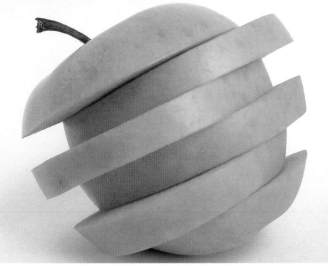

Vegetables

The following are No-Check vegetables and may be eaten freely at any time:

asparagus, aubergine, baby sweetcorn, bamboo shoots, beansprouts, beetroot, broccoli, Brussels sprouts, cabbage, calabrese, carrots, cauliflower, celeriac, celery, chard, chicory, Chinese leaves, christophene, courgettes, cress/mustard & cress, cucumber, endive, fennel, green beans, Jerusalem artichokes, kale, leeks, lettuce, mangetout, marrow, mooli, mushrooms, okra, onions, pak choi/bok choi, peppers, pumpkin, radishes, salsify, spinach, spring greens, squash, sugar snap peas, swede, tomatoes, turnips, water chestnuts, watercress

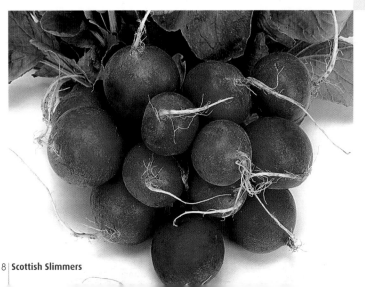

Hectic Life

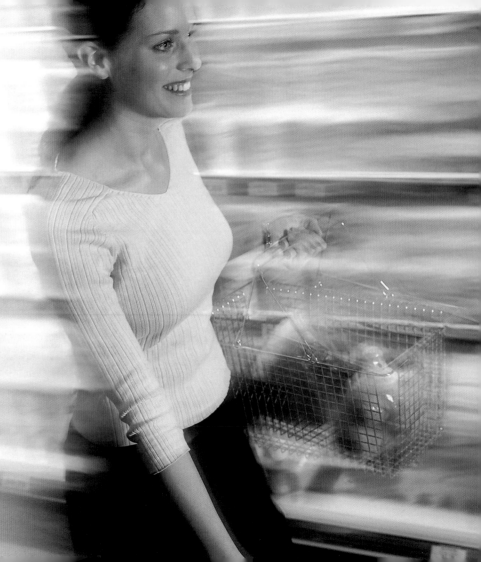

Nowadays, life can be pretty hectic with little time available for cooking complicated meals. This plan shows how easy it can be to mix and match healthier convenience foods with fresh foods in order to produce quick and easy meals that are nutritious, delicious and won't leave you standing in the kitchen for hours on end.

In this plan we give examples of three meals a day and give the total number of Checks spent on meals. We've also included Every Day Bonus foods – so all you have to do is add your favourite Essential Extras up to your daily Check allowance.

Time-saver tips

Make the most of pre-prepared fresh vegetables and salads and frozen vegetables. You'll be more likely to include plenty of veg if you don't have to spend a lot of time peeling and chopping. Individual microwavable bags of vegetables are very convenient when cooking for one. Frozen cooked rice is another valuable timesaver.

If you rely too heavily on convenience foods, you could be low on fibre. Your five-a-day servings of fruit and veg supply about half your daily requirement. Get the remainder from high-fibre foods such as wholemeal bread, wholemeal pasta, brown rice, wholegrain cereals, peas, beans, lentils, jacket and new potatoes.

Individual portion packs save weighing time – and temptation! You can also save weighing by looking at the portion weight you need, and looking at the weight on the can, jar or pack. Is it about a half or a quarter or a third of the pack? With the exception of very high-calorie foods such as fats, oils, fatty meats, cream and full-fat cheese, a few grams more or less will make very little difference.

If you choose a ready-meal, select from a "healthy" range. In addition to having a lower Check and fat gram value, they are usually lower in salt than the equivalent from a supermarket standard range. Canned foods can also be very high in salt, so go for reduced-salt or no-added-salt options whenever you can.

Make the most of your microwave! Short cooking times mean that, not only do you get your dinner on the table much more quickly, but more vitamins are preserved. Fish and vegetables are particularly good in the microwave.

Quickly stir-frying veg also preserves texture, colour and nutrients.

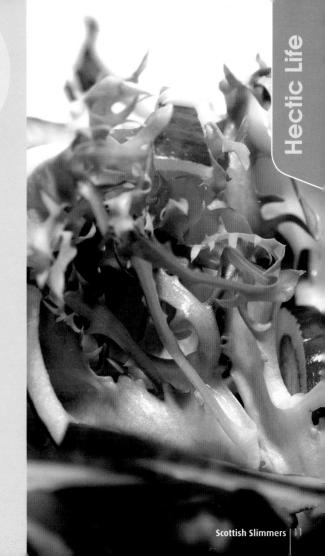

Monday

 average

EDB 150ml skimmed use in drinks

8 **1** Cereal pack

40-45g individual pack any Nestlé wholegrain cereal plus 150ml skimmed milk.

EDB 2 satsumas

10 **5** Tuna salad sandwich

Drain 85-100g can tuna in brine and mix with 1 dspn low-calorie mayonnaise. Fill 2 medium slices wholemeal bread with the mixture and No-Check salad. (Or any up-to-300-calories supermarket sandwich).

EDB 100g pot diet fromage frais

15 **9** Pasta bolognese

Boil 60g pasta shapes. Microwave 170g pouch Dolmio Minced Beef Bolognese. Serve over drained pasta and top with 1 dspn grated parmesan or half-fat cheese. Accompany with No-Check salad.

EDB 1 peach or nectarine

Total meal Checks
33 **15**

Don't forget to add your Essential Extras!

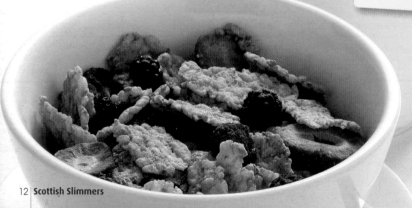

Tuesday

EDB 150ml skimmed milk for use in drinks

8 **4** Toast & marmalade

2 medium slices wholemeal toast, 1 tsp low-fat spread and 2 tsp reduced-sugar marmalade.

EDB 1 apple

12 **14** Crispbreads & pâté

85g (half 170g pack) low-fat pâté, 4 Ryvita Original or Dark Rye. Serve with cherry tomatoes and salad leaves.

EDB 100g pot diet fromage frais

15 **5** Saucy fish & rice

Boil 60g rice (or microwave 130g frozen rice). Boil or microwave 1 individual portion Young's Cod in Butter Sauce and serve over rice together with 2 tbsp peas, broccoli or other No-Check vegetables.

EDB 2 large plums

Total meal Checks
35 **23**

Don't forget to add your Essential Extras!

Wednesday

EDB 150ml skimmed milk for use in drinks

8 **1** Cereal pack

40-45g individual pack any Nestlé wholegrain cereal plus 150ml skimmed milk.

EDB 2 small kiwi fruits

12 **14** Crispbreads & pâté

85g (half 170g pack) low-fat pâté, 4 Ryvita Original or Dark Rye. Serve with cherry tomatoes and salad leaves.

EDB 1 peach or nectarine

15 **8** Steam Fresh Thai

Microwave 1 pack Birds Eye Steam Fresh Thai Chicken with Steamed Rice according to instructions and serve with additional No-Check vegetables. Or, use No-Check vegetables to make soup for a starter. (nb: Birds Eye have lowered the salt content of all their meals.)

EDB 100g pot diet fromage frais

Total meal Checks
35 **23**
Don't forget to add your Essential Extras!

Thursday

EDB 150ml skimmed milk for use in drinks

8 **4** Toast & marmalade

2 medium slices wholemeal toast, 1 tsp low-fat spread and 2 tsp reduced-sugar marmalade.

EDB 2 large plums

11 **7** Chicken tikka wrap

Place salad leaves and cucumber strips on 1 flour tortilla or wrap. Top with 100g chicken tikka mini fillets (or other flavour) and 1 dspn fat-free natural fromage frais. Roll up.

EDB 1 apple

15 **14** Simple salmon

Microwave 125g salmon fillet, lightly seasoned and sprinkled with lemon juice. Serve with 200g new potatoes, green beans, broccoli or other No-Check vegetables. (nb: cook double the quantity of potatoes and save half for tomorrow.)

EDB 100g pot diet fromage frais

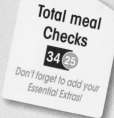

Total meal Checks
34 **25**
Don't forget to add your Essential Extras!

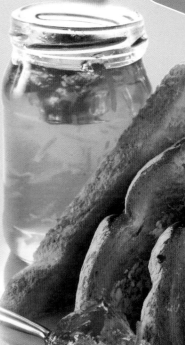

Friday

EDB 150ml skimmed milk for use in drinks

8 **1** Cereal pack

40-45g individual pack any Nestlé wholegrain cereal plus 150ml skimmed milk.

EDB 2 satsumas

11 **7** Chicken tikka wrap

Place salad leaves and cucumber strips on 1 flour tortilla or wrap. Top with 100g chicken tikka mini fillets (or other flavour) and 1 dspn fat-free natural fromage frais. Roll up.

EDB 125g pot diet yoghurt

12 **6** Sausage, peppers & new potato pan-fry

Grill 2 Wall's Lean Recipe sausages, then cut into slices. Cook 1 sliced onion and handful of frozen mixed peppers in pan sprayed with oil. Remove. Re-spray pan. Cover base with 200g sliced cooked new potatoes. Brown underneath, turn over and brown other side. Return vegetables and sausages to pan with a pinch of chilli. Heat through.

EDB 1 peach or nectarine

Total meal Checks
31 **14**

Don't forget to add your Essential Extras!

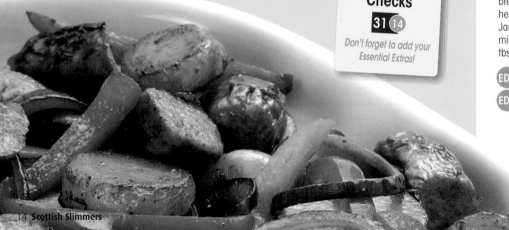

Saturday

EDB 150ml skimmed milk for use in drinks

6 **5** Cheese on toast

Place 30g sliced half-fat cheddar and thin slices tomato on 1 medium slice toast. Grill until cheese melts.

12 **5** Ham salad pannini/baguette

Warm a 85-100g pannini in the oven. Split and fill with No-Check salad and 4 wafer-thin slices ham. Alternatively, use 100g French baguette.

16 **5** Jerk chicken & wedges

Microwave 275g potato. Cut cooked potato into 8 wedges, spray with oil and brown in pre-heated hot oven approximately 25 minutes. Spray 1 skinless chicken breast with oil and grill 25 minutes under moderate heat, turning half-way. Sprinkle over ½ tsp Schwartz Jamaican Jerk Grill & Sizzle and return to low grill 1-2 minutes. Serve chicken with the wedges, 2 rounded tbsp peas or sweetcorn and grilled tomatoes.

EDB 1 medium banana or mango

EDB 125g pot diet yoghurt

Total meal Checks
34 **15**

Don't forget to add your Essential Extras!

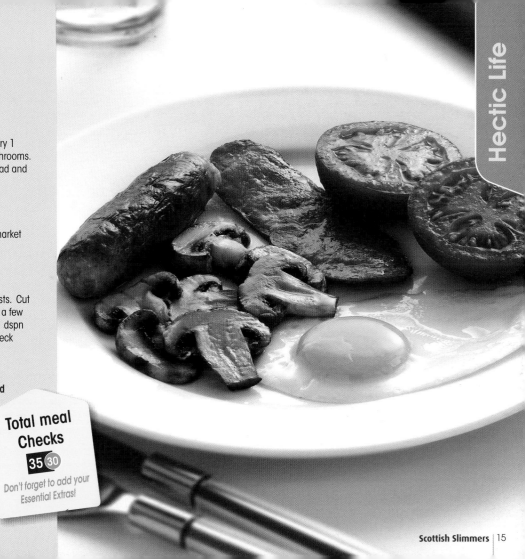

Sunday

EDB 150ml skimmed milk for use in drinks

14 **14** Late riser brunch

Grill 2 Wall's Lean Recipe Sausages. Poach or dry-fry 1 medium egg. Serve with grilled tomatoes and mushrooms. 1 medium slice wholemeal toast, 1 tsp low-fat spread and 2 tsp reduced-sugar marmalade.

5 **4** Choc drink & cake slice

average

1 sachet High Lights Chocolate Drink and 1 supermarket "healthy" cake slice.

16 **12** Pork medallions

Ovenbake 150g frozen weight McCain's Home Roasts. Cut 100g pork fillet/tenderloin into thin slices and cook a few minutes in pan sprayed with oil. Make gravy from 1 dspn Oxo or Bisto Best gravy granules. Serve with No-Check vegetables and 1 dspn apple or cranberry sauce.

EDB 1 large cooking apple, baked or microwaved with pinch of spice.

EDB 125g pot diet yoghurt

Total meal Checks
35 **30**
Don't forget to add your Essential Extras!

Essential Extras for a hectic life!

Choose Extras up to the value of your daily allowance.

1 small slice bread	2	0.5
1 medium slice bread	3	1
1 thick slice bread	4	1
50g bread roll	5	1
50g crusty bread	5	2
1 Ryvita Original or Dark Rye	1	0

1 tsp low-fat spread	1	2
1 tsp oil	1.5	4
1 dspn low-calorie mayonnaise	1	3
1 dspn Oxo or Bisto Best gravy granules	1	0

50g pack ready-to-eat apricots or prunes	3	0
1 rounded tbsp dried fruit	2	0
Supermarket "healthy" cake slice, average	3.5	2
Danone Shape Fruit Juice Mousse	5	3
M&S COU Café Mocha Dessert 115g	5	3
150g 99% fat-free Mullerice, flavoured	5	1.5

Burger King LA Flame Grilled Chicken Sandwich	11	4
McDonald's Grilled Chicken Caeser Salad, no dressing	9	9
Starbucks Cappuccino, skimmed, tall	3	0
Subway, 6g or less fat, Beef or Turkey sub	11	4
Subway, 6g or less fat, Veggie Delite sub	8	3

Low-calorie cup soup, average	2	1
High Lights Chocolate Drink	1.5	1.5
125ml glass of wine	4	0
275ml Bacardi Breezer Half Sugar	5	0

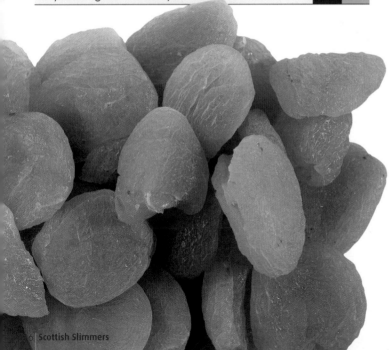

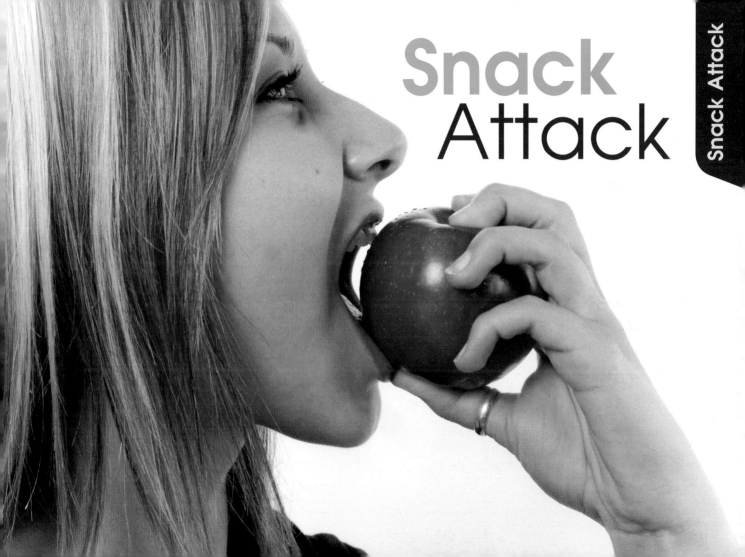

Snack
Attack

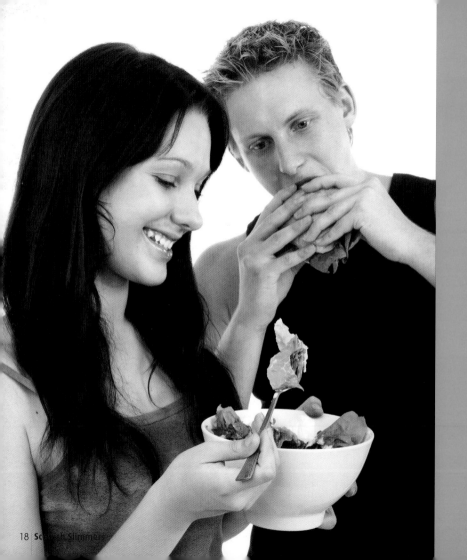

Eating small, regular meals and snacks helps prevent dips in blood sugar levels. These can leave you feeling faint and tempted to eat the first thing you can lay your hands on!

This plan shows how you can split your daily Checks allowance into 6 or 7 meals/snacks a day.

It is based on an average of 40 Checks per day with Every Day Bonus foods included. If you are allowed more than this, you can add even more Essential Extras up to your daily allowance. Remember that Essential Extras can be used to increase portion sizes within a meal as well as for between meal snacks. Feel free to swap your favourite meals and snacks up to the same Check values as those shown.

Meals and snacks may be eaten in any order.

Our recommendation is always that you eat at a time that best suits your lifestyle. When you eat pales into insignificance compared to how much you eat. It is true that if you are active soon after eating, you will burn off calories before they have a chance to settle as fat, but if you have eaten more calories than you can use up over the next few hours, they will be stored as fat anyway.

No matter at what time you sleep or eat, there are still 24 hours in your day, so if you are a shift worker, simply plan to have your whole day's allowance any time between midnight and midnight.

If your shift goes across midnight, this might mean you pack up and take the last meal or snack from one day, and one or two from the next day. You can use the table below to plan when you will eat on your various shift patterns.

Meal or Snack	Shift 1 Meal Times	Shift 2 Meals Times	Shift 3 Meal Times
1			
2			
3			
4			
5			
6			
(7)			

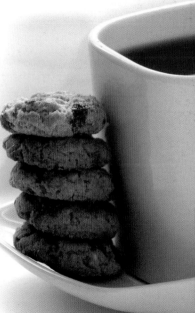

Monday

EDB 150ml skimmed milk for use in drinks.

EDB 1 medium banana

EDB 125g pot diet yoghurt

6 8 Boiled egg & soldiers

1 medium boiled egg, 1 small slice wholemeal toast, 1 tsp low-fat spread.

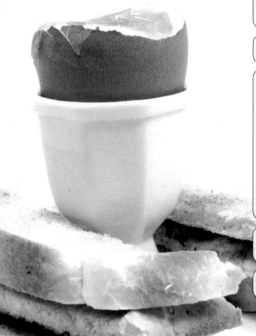

12 11 Oatcakes & soft cheese

3 oatcakes with 100g Philadelphia Extra Light Soft Cheese, cherry tomatoes and celery sticks. 1 apple.

4 0 2 rounded tbsp raisins or sultanas

11 6 Warm chicken, bacon & crouton salad

Grill 1 chicken breast and 2 bacon medallions. Toast 1 small slice wholemeal bread. Chop bacon and chicken and cut toast into cubes. Sprinkle oil-free vinaigrette onto shredded lettuce and tomato wedges. Mix with chicken, bacon and toast and sprinkle with 1 dspn grated parmesan cheese.

2 2 1 small level scoop ice cream with sugar-free jelly.

4 5 24g pack Walker's Lights crisps

Tuesday

EDB 150ml skimmed milk for use in drinks.

6 2 Instant porridge

1 sachet Oatso-Simple Original made according to instructions with skimmed milk.

7 4 50-60g roll filled with 1 tsp low-fat spread, 2 slices wafer-thin ham and salad.

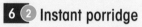

10 4 Soup & salad roll

295g can low-calorie soup (up to 100 calories). 50-60g roll filled with salad.

EDB 125g pot diet yoghurt

14 7 Cottage pie

Brown 100g lean mince with chopped onion. Drain any surplus fat. Add thinly sliced/chopped carrot and 150ml water. Simmer covered until carrots are tender. Stir in 1 dspn low-fat gravy granules. Place in ovenproof dish. Boil 200g potato plus turnip/swede or carrot and mash with a little skimmed milk. Spread over mince and brown in a moderate oven or under the grill. Serve with No-Check vegetables.

EDB 1 large cooking apple, baked, stewed or microwaved with a pinch of spice.

3 1 Alpen Light cereal bar

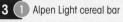

Wednesday

EDB 150ml skimmed milk for use in drinks.

6 **2** **Mushrooms on toast**

Serve grilled mushrooms on 3 small slices toast.

3 **1** 1 Alpen Light cereal bar

EDB 2 satsumas

9 **10** **Salmon salad (1)**

Serve half of 185-215g can pink salmon with a large No-Check salad, 1 dspn low-calorie mayonnaise and 1 small slice bread.

EDB 125g pot diet yoghurt

EDB 1 peach or nectarine

14 **11** **Tasty chicken & jacket**

Grill or bake 1 Birds Eye Chicken Chargrill, Cracked Pepper Chicken, Thai Chicken or Tikka Chicken. Bake or microwave 200g potato in its jacket and serve with No-Check vegetables or salad.

9 **10** **Salmon salad (2)**

Serve remaining half of 185-215g can pink salmon with a large No-Check salad, 1 dspn low-calorie mayonnaise and 1 small slice bread.

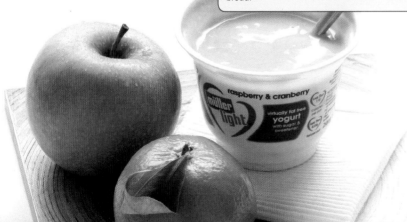

Thursday

EDB 150ml skimmed milk for use in drinks.

6 **7** **Ham 'n' egg**

Place 1 wafer-thin slice ham on 1 small slice toast. Top with 1 poached or microwaved egg.

EDB 2 satsumas

10 **10** **Oatcakes & soft cheese**

3 oatcakes with 100g Philadelphia Extra Light Soft Cheese, cherry tomatoes and celery sticks.

EDB 1 apple or pear
2 **0** 1 dspn raisins or sultanas

13 **2** **Cod Portugaise**

Par-boil 200g chunks of potato with sliced peppers and onions. Drain, reserving liquid. Return to pan and add 200g canned tomatoes, crushed garlic, good pinch chilli, ½ stock cube and 1 tbsp white wine. Simmer 10 minutes. Add 175g cod and simmer 5-10 minutes adding liquid if required. Garnish with chopped parsley.

9 **3** **Beans on Toast**

Serve 200g can reduced-sugar-and-salt baked beans on 2 small slices toast. Top with 20g grated half-fat cheese from EDB allowance.

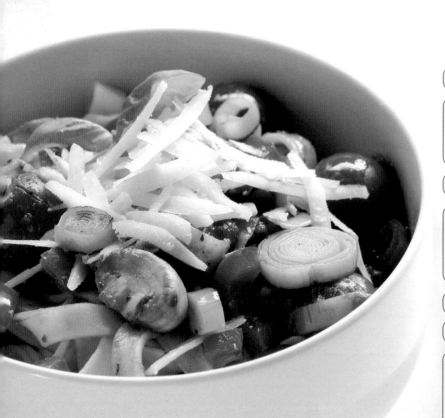

Friday

6 **8** **Boiled egg & soldiers**

1 medium boiled egg, 1 small slice wholemeal toast,
1 tsp low-fat spread.

EDB 1 apple

9 **6** **Ham triple-decker**

Make a triple-decker sandwich from 3 small slices bread, 1 tsp
low-fat spread, 4 wafer-thin slices ham and plenty of No-Check
salad.

EDB 125g pot diet yoghurt

EDB 85g grapes

12 **6** **Leek & mushroom tagliatelle**

Boil 75g tagliatelle. Fry chopped leek in pan sprayed with oil.
Add chopped pepper, mushrooms, 1 dspn tomato purée, 200g
canned tomatoes, pinch mixed herbs and ½ Oxo vegetable cube.
Simmer 10 minutes, stirring frequently. Serve topped with 2 dspn
grated parmesan.

4 **4** 2 small level scoops ice cream and sugar-free jelly.

8 **5** 125ml glass of wine and 24g pack Walker's Lights crisps.

Saturday

EDB 150ml skimmed milk for use in drinks.

6 **2** Instant porridge

1 sachet Oatso-Simple Original made according to instructions with skimmed milk.

EDB 2 satsumas

12 **8** BLT

Toast 4 small slices of bread and grill 2 bacon medallions. Make into 2 sandwiches with lettuce, tomato and 2 tsp low-calorie mayonnaise.

EDB 1 nectarine or peach

EDB 75g Total 0% fat Greek yoghurt

13 **3** Chilli prawns

Chop spring onion, green pepper, red pepper and 1 clove garlic. Mix with 1 dspn grated ginger. Cook 1-2 minutes in pan sprayed with oil. Add 150g prawns, 1 dspn tomato purée, 1 tsp chilli sauce, ½ tsp sugar, dash of vinegar, salt and pepper. Stir-fry until prawns are well coated. Serve with 45g dry weight boiled rice or noodles.

8 **5** 125ml glass of wine and 24g pack Walker's Lights crisps.

Sunday

EDB 150ml skimmed milk for use in drinks.

6 **7** Bacon & waffle grill

Grill 2 bacon medallions, 1 potato waffle, mushrooms and tomatoes.

3 **1** 1 Alpen Light cereal bar

8 **8** Cheese toast salad

Prepare a salad of No-Check vegetables. Slice 40g half-fat cheese and place on 2 small slices toast. Grill until cheese melts and serve with the salad.

EDB 1 medium banana

EDB 75g Total 0% fat Greek yoghurt

15 **10** Hotpot

Cube 125g lean beef or lamb. Place in casserole dish with sliced onion, celery and carrot. Coat with 1 tbsp flour. Crumble over 1 Oxo cube. Pour in 200ml water. Slice 175g potato over mixture, cover tightly. Cook in moderate oven approximately 1½ hours. Serve with No-Check vegetables.

6 **2** Danone Shape Goodies Trifle

4 **5** 17.5g Cadburys Dairy Milk Under 99 Calories.

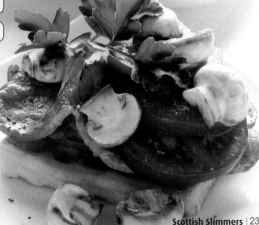

Essential Extras

Extras have been included in the Snack Attack plan – if you are allowed, you can choose even more from the list below up to your allowance.

1 small slice bread	2	0.5
1 medium slice bread	3	1
1 Paterson's oatcake	2	2
150g potato	4	0
200g potato	6	0.5
30g dry weight pasta or rice	4	0.5

Fox's Officially Low Fat Cereal Bar	3	0.5
26g pack Scottish Slimmers Mini Cookies	5	5
Mr Kipling Delightful Chocolate Slice	4	2
25g pack Jacob's Thai Bites	4	1

No-Check Winter Vegetable Soup

4 servings

Place 3-4 diced medium carrots, 150g diced turnip, 1 large chopped onion and 3 sticks sliced celery in a large saucepan with 2 tbsp water. Bring to the boil, then cover and sweat gently 10 minutes. Add 900ml chicken or vegetable stock and simmer covered 15 minutes. Serve chunky or crush vegetables and garnish with a little finely chopped parsley.

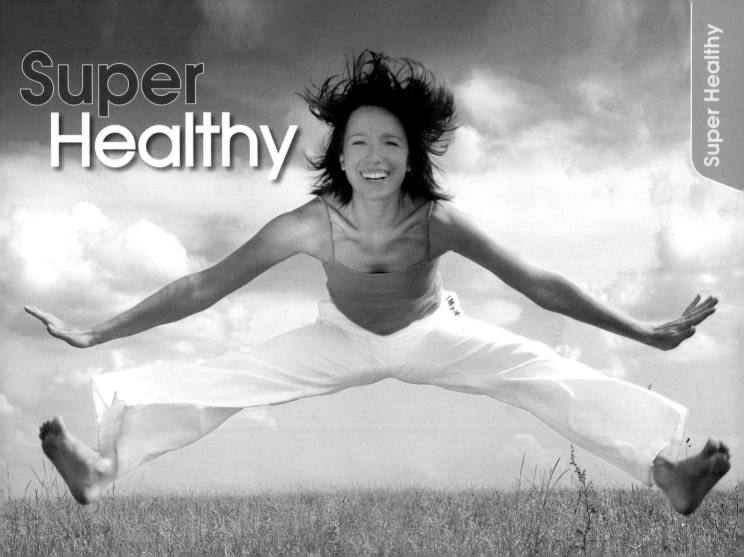

Super
Healthy

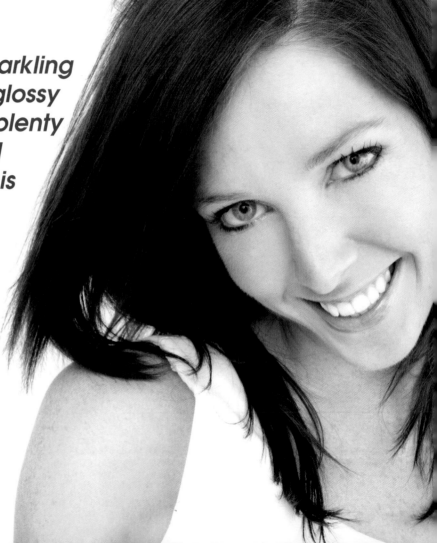

If you are looking for sparkling eyes, smooth skin and glossy hair, you'll need to eat plenty of foods rich in essential nutrients. And this plan is choc-full of them!

In addition, many of the foods that help you look good are also those most likely to protect your health and lower the risk of getting serious diseases, as well as keeping you looking and feeling youthful longer.

For each day we have suggested three meals and show the total Checks for these meals. In addition, you should have your usual Every Day Bonus foods, and also add Essential Extras up to your daily Check allowance.

Go green!

Leafy greens, especially broccoli and spinach, contain a host of compounds including anti-oxidant vitamins A and E. They are also high in folates important in pregnancy. Folates also lower levels of homocysteine which are associated with heart disease.

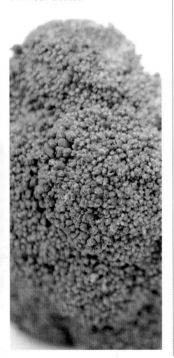

Carrots & co

Caretenoids are found in many orange-coloured fruits and veg such as carrots, pumpkin, butternut squash, red and orange peppers, sweet potatoes, apricots and mangos. They are thought to reduce risk of cancer, help protect skin and eyes from the effects of ultra-violet light and reduce the risk of cataract and age-related macular disease. Lycopene, another caretenoid, found in tomatoes, watermelon, pink grapefruit, papaya and guavas, may also act like a sun-screen and is thought to reduce risk of prostate cancer. More lycopene is released when tomatoes are cooked – think pasta sauce!

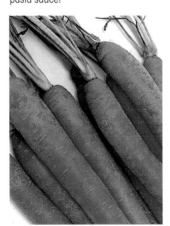

Very berry

The anthocyanins in blueberries, cranberries, raspberries, blackberries, red and blackcurrants help produce collagen for great skin. Blueberries, may slow down age-related diseases such as dementia and Alzheimers, and along with cranberries are helpful in treating urinary tract infections. Similar compounds are also found in red and black grapes, red wine, pomegranates, aubergines, red onions, red cabbage and black and green tea.

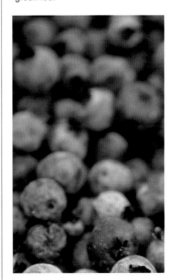

Citrus fruits

Well known for being a brilliant source of anti-oxidant vitamin C. Substances in the pith and peel of citrus fruits may prevent cells from mutating – often the first steps in cancer and degenerative diseases. A great excuse for eating reduced-sugar chunky marmalade, grating zest into recipes or slicing kumquats into your fruit salad.

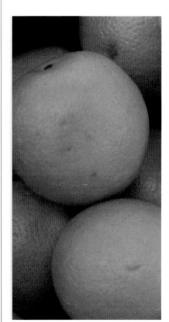

Monday

8 **Porridge & berries**

Make porridge from 40g oats, 150ml skimmed milk and water as required. Serve topped with a handful of your favourite fresh or defrosted frozen berries.

12 **8** **Cheese & fruit plate**

60g half-fat cheese, or 3 Baby Bel Light Minis, 1 apple, 1 kiwi fruit, 1 satsuma and a small bunch of red or black grapes.

16 **9** **Pasta with peppers & mushrooms**

Brown 85g extra lean mince. Add a good handful of frozen mixed sliced peppers, 2-3 sliced mushrooms and cook until peppers are just tender. Add 200g low-fat pasta sauce and warm through. Serve with 60g dry weight, boiled wholemeal pasta.

Total meal Checks **36** **20**

Don't forget to add Every Day Bonus foods and Essential Extras!

Oats and wholegrains

Oats contain soluble fibre which helps lower cholesterol and keeps hunger at bay. Wholegrains help prevent constipation and lower risk of stroke and coronary artery disease. They are also rich in B vitamins which release energy from food.

Tuesday

8 **2** **Muesli or Kashi**

40g no-added-sugar muesli or Kashi Original Seven Grains cereal with 150ml skimmed milk.

13 **20** **Mackerel salad**

Prepare a large No-Check salad including some dark leafy greens such as Cos, Romaine, Little Gem or Rocket. Add either 75g smoked mackerel fillet or 120g can mackerel fillets in tomato sauce. Serve with 1 medium slice wholemeal bread.

14 **Lemon chicken with confetti rice**

Marinate 1 chicken breast in 1 tsp soy sauce, squeeze of lemon juice, 1 tsp grated lemon zest and 1 crushed garlic clove. Bake in a moderate oven or grill approximately 20 minutes. Boil 60g rice. Drain and stir in chopped peppers, spring onion and parsley.

Total meal Checks **35** **24**

Don't forget to add Every Day Bonus foods and Essential Extras!

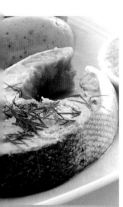

Oily fish

Is great for heart-healthy omega 3s. These amazing oils may also have a role in preventing breast and colon cancers, ADHD, dementia and Alzheimers, joint pain associated with arthritis, brittle nails, weak hair and dry skin! Oily fish such as salmon, mackerel, trout, sardines and pilchards are also a good source of vitamin D which plays an important role in bone formation.

Wednesday

8 **9 Cranberry juice & peanut butter toast**

100ml Ocean Spray Cranberry Juice Light. Spread 2 tsp peanut butter on 1 medium slice wholemeal toast.

12 11 Sunflower salad

Mix 150g cooked weight, cold wholemeal pasta (made from 60g dry), 2-3 sliced raw mushrooms and 4 halved cherry tomatoes. Dress with 1 tsp olive oil mixed with 1 dspn balsamic vinegar and scatter with 1 tbsp sunflower or pumpkin seeds.

16 5 Pork escalopes with sweet potato wedges

Boil 250g sweet potatoes until just tender, cut into wedges, spray with oil and brown in a hot oven. Grill or pan-fry in spray oil 115g pork escalopes. Serve with 2 tbsp peas and other No-Check vegetables.

Total meal Checks 36 25

Don't forget to add Every Day Bonus foods and Essential Extras!

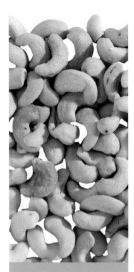

Nuts & seeds

Are the best source of vitamin E which has anti-inflammatory properties, and are also rich in minerals such as zinc (especially pumpkin seeds), iron, copper and magnesium. Nuts containing a higher percentage of better-for-you monounsaturated fats include peanuts, almonds, hazelnuts, macadamias and pecans.

Thursday

7 **6 Pink Grapefruit, oatcakes & cheese**

½ large pink grapefruit. 2 oatcakes with 30g extra light soft cheese.

12 3 Chicken & chutney pitta

Cut a medium wholemeal pitta bread into 2 pockets. Line with lettuce and fill with 75g cooked chicken or turkey breast and 2 tsp mango chutney or cranberry sauce.

14 11 Chickpea & spinach curry

Cook 1 small sliced onion and crushed garlic in oil-sprayed pan. Add 1 tbsp medium curry paste. Stir in 200g canned tomatoes, 4 rounded tbsp canned chickpeas and some fresh or frozen spinach. Bring to simmering point, cover and leave 20 minutes. Season with salt, pepper and lemon juice. Serve with 50g dry weight, boiled rice or 1 wholemeal pitta bread.

Total meal Checks 33 20

Don't forget to add Every Day Bonus foods and Essential Extras!

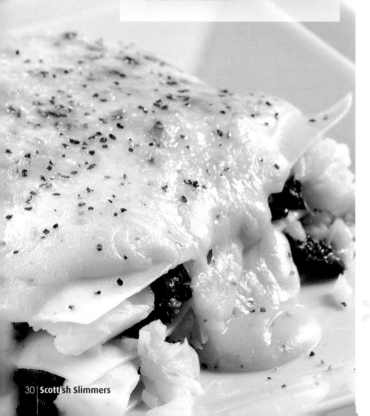

Lean meats & white fish

Excellent sources of protein for repair of cells, and zinc for wound healing and production of sex hormones. Lean red meats are the best source of iron to prevent fatigue. White fish also contains iodine needed for thyroid hormones which control metabolism.

 Probiotic drink, toast & marmalade

1 small bottle Yakult or Actimel Light. 1 medium slice wholemeal toast spread with 1 tsp oilive oil spread and 2 tsp reduced-sugar marmalade.

 Carrot & coriander soup with roll

300ml fresh carrot & coriander soup (e.g. New Covent Garden), 1 wholemeal roll filled with 1 tsp oilive oil spread and No-Check salad.

 Florentine Lasagne

Microwave 170g Birds Eye Cod Steak in Butter Sauce. Cook 150g frozen spinach and drain well. Boil 3 lasagne sheets, drain and place 1 on a plate. Cover with half the spinach. Remove half the fish leaving sauce in pack. Place over spinach. Repeat layers. Top with lasagne sheet, butter sauce and 1 tbsp parmesan. Microwave 1 minute to heat through.

Total meal Checks

* Don't forget to add Every Day Bonus foods and Essential Extras!

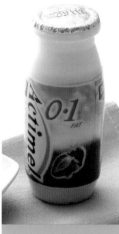

Yoghurt

As well as being a terrific source of protein and calcium, bio yoghurts and pro-biotic cultured milk drinks can encourage friendly bacteria and also help decrease yeast infections.

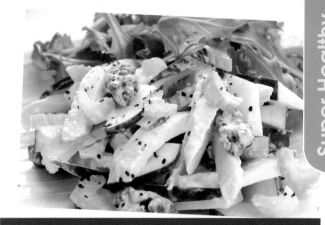
Saturday

7 **1** ## Banana, yoghurt & wheatgerm

Slice 1 medium banana and top with 125g pot virtually-fat-free bio yoghurt and 1 tbsp wheatgerm.

11 **3** ## Beans on toast

Warm a 200g can of reduced-sugar-and-salt baked beans and serve on 2 medium slices wholemeal toast.

16 **8** ## Sesame chicken with garlic greens

Marinate 1 skinless chicken breast in 1 tsp light soy sauce, 1 tsp dry sherry and pinch of ground ginger at least 15 minutes. Heat 1 tsp oil and stir-fry chicken 5 minutes. Add 2 sliced mushrooms and cook 2 minutes. Add 1 tsp sesame seeds and cook 1 minute. Remove from pan. Add crushed garlic clove and heat. Stir in 100g pak choi or shredded Savoy cabbage and 1 dspn water and stir 1-2 minutes. Sprinkle with soy. Serve with 60g dry weight, noodles.

Total meal Checks **34** **12**

Don't forget to add Every Day Bonus foods and Essential Extras!

Pulses

All types of peas, beans and lentils are high in fibre and help stabilise blood sugar levels as they have a low GI rating.

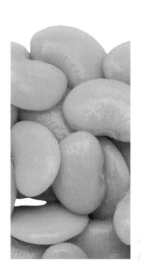

Sunday

8 **8** ## Juice, egg & toast

200ml Ocean Spray Cranberry Juice Light. 1 large Columbus egg (with Omega 3), boiled and 1 medium slice wholemeal toast.

12 **9** ## Chicken & walnut salad

Toss 85g cooked chopped chicken, 1 cored and chopped apple, 1 small sliced stick celery and 3 roughly chopped walnut halves in 2 rounded tbsp low-fat natural yoghurt. Season with lemon juice, salt and black pepper.

16 **7** ## Steak & jacket

Grill 150g lean steak. Ovenbake or microwave 200g potato in its jacket. Serve with 2 tbsp peas, grilled tomatoes and mushrooms, and No-Check salad.

Total meal Checks **36** **24**

Don't forget to add Every Day Bonus foods and Essential Extras!

Super Healthy Essential Extras

100g Shearway frozen Blueberries or Black Forest Fruits	2	0
1 large mango or medium papaya	4	0

30g porridge oats	4	2
1 slice Burgen Wholegrain & Cranberry bread	4	2
30g Kashi Original Seven Grains	4	1
1 Ryvita Pumpkin Seeds & Oats	2	1
1 Ryvita Sunflower Seeds & Oats	1.5	1

1 Paterson's Oatcake	2	2
1 large Columbus Egg with Omega 3	4	7

26g pack Scottish Slimmers Syrupy Oat Cookies	5	5
1 Jordan's Crunchy Honey & Almond Bar	5	6
1 Quaker Oat Bar	6	3.5
25g pumpkin seeds	6	12
25g The Food Doctor Original Seed Mix	5	11
25g peanuts and raisins	4	7
50g ready-to-eat apricots	3	0
50g ready-to-eat prunes	3	0

1 cup of green tea	No-Check	
125ml glass red wine	4	0
250ml Innocent Cranberries & Raspberries Smoothie	4	0
100ml bottle Vie Shots	3	0
330ml bottle Pomegreat Pomegranate Juice Drink	6	0

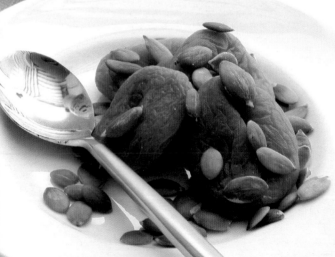

Go
Veggie

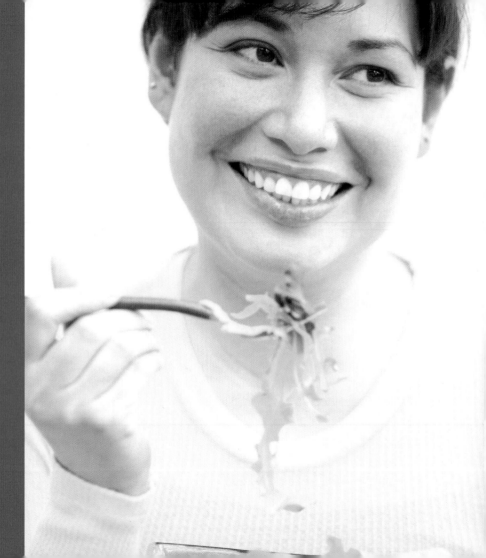

Being vegetarian has never been simpler – nor tastier! This meat-free plan can be enjoyed by vegetarians and non-vegetarians alike.

For each day we have suggested three meals and show the total Checks for these meals. In addition, you should have your usual **Every Day Bonus** foods, and also add **Essential Extras** up to your daily Check allowance.

The key to a great vegetarian diet is to ensure you include lots of variety in your meals and snacks. Here are a few pointers.

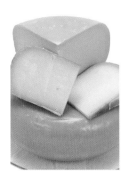

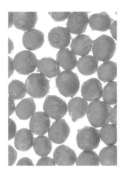

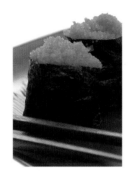

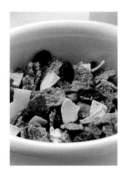

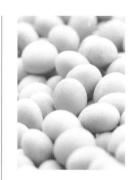

Dairy produce such as milk, yoghurt, cheese and eggs provide top quality protein as well as providing calcium for strong bones and teeth – so don't forget to always have at least your Every Day Bonus allowance. Calcium-enriched soy milk can be used if preferred.

Soya products and Quorn also provide top quality protein. Beans, peas and lentils also provide good amounts of protein with the quality being improved if they are mixed either with nuts and seeds, or cereals and grains such as breads, pasta, rice, bulghur wheat, millet and couscous.

Vitamin B12 is very important for red blood cell formation and the manufacture of genetic material but is not generally found in plant foods. Some sources are fortified cereals, yeast extract (e.g. Marmite), Quorn, seaweeds such as sushi nori, or the friendly bacteria in beer!

Although many vegetables and pulses contain iron, the type of iron they contain is not as easily absorbed as iron from meat. You can improve absorption by eating it with something rich in vitamin C such as having a glass of orange juice with an iron fortified breakfast cereal. Avoid drinking tea at the same meal as the tannin prevents iron from being absorbed.

Zinc and other minerals are often found in the beans, peas, nuts, seeds and dairy produce eaten for protein.

Monday

8 **2** Greek yoghurt, banana
& chopped dates

Chop 1 medium banana and 2 dates. Mix
together and top with 2 tbsp 0% fat Greek yoghurt
and 1 tsp chopped mixed nuts.

10 **11** Egg & cress sandwich

Fill 2 medium slices bread with 1 sliced hard-
boiled egg, 1 dspn low-calorie mayonnaise or
salad cream and cress or shredded lettuce.

16 **14** Spinach &
ricotta tortellini

Boil 150g fresh spinach & ricotta tortellini/
tortelloni or ravioli. Warm 125g (quarter of 500g
jar) Dolmio Light Pasta Sauce, serve over pasta
and top with 1 tbsp grated parmesan or half-fat
cheese. Serve with a No-Check salad on the side.

Total meal Checks **34** **27**

*Don't forget to add Every Day Bonus foods
and Essential Extras!*

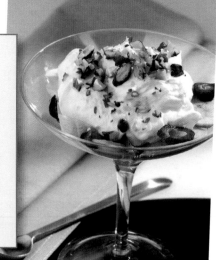

Tuesday

8 **6** My mate

2 medium slices bread or toast each spread
with 1 tsp low-fat spread and Marmite or other
yeast extract to taste.

12 **8** Roasted vegetable wrap

Cut 1 pepper, 1 courgette, 1 small onion and
2 tomatoes into chunks. Spray with oil and
roast in a hot oven until starting to char. (Can
be prepared in advance.) Spread the hot or
cold vegetables over 2 flour tortillas. Top each
with 1 tbsp fat-free natural fromage frais and
roll up.

14 **5** Sausage & mash

Grill 2 Quorn sausages. Boil 275g potato and
mash with a little skimmed milk. Slice 1 onion
and cook in pan sprayed with oil. Make gravy
from 1 dspn Oxo vegetable gravy granules.
Mix with onions and pour over sausages.
Serve with cabbage and carrots or other No-
Check vegetables.

Total meal Checks **34** **19**

*Don't forget to add Every Day Bonus foods
and Essential Extras*

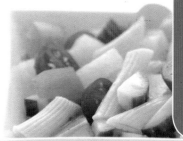

Wednesday

8 2 Juice & cereal

100ml unsweetened orange juice. 30g cereal (preferably fortified with iron and vitamin B12), 150ml skimmed milk.

11 8 Pasta salad mix

Mix 75g cooked weight pasta or rice (from 30g dry weight) with 30g Edam or 45g half-fat cheddar, 1 chopped pineapple ring, 2 tbsp sweetcorn, chopped tomato, onion, cucumber and oil-free vinaigrette.

15 5 Vegetable chilli

Soften 1 small sliced onion and crushed garlic in 1 tsp olive oil. Add 200g canned tomatoes, 1 tbsp tomato purée, good handful sliced peppers, 200g can drained kidney beans, pinch of cumin and chilli powder to taste. Simmer until vegetables are tender. Season to taste and serve either with 60g dry weight boiled rice or 275g potato microwaved or jacket baked.

Total meal Checks 34 15

Don't forget to add Every Day Bonus foods and Essential Extras!

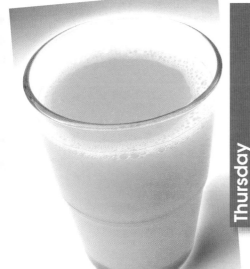

Thursday

8 7 Juice, egg & toast

100ml unsweetened orange juice. 1 medium egg boiled or poached. 1 medium slice bread or toast.

11 12 Houmous & pitta

Serve 1 medium pitta bread with 2 rounded tbsp reduced-fat houmous and No-Check salad.

14 8 Cheesy hash

Sauté 1 chopped onion in spray oil until transparent. Add 275g cooked potato and some cooked carrot, turnip/swede or other No-Check vegetables. Add 30g grated half-fat cheddar – mash together if preferred. Sprinkle with a further 30g grated half-fat cheddar and brown under grill. Serve with No-Check salad or grilled tomatoes.

Total meal Checks 33 27

Don't forget to add Every Day Bonus foods and Essential Extras!

8 ② Porridge with raisins

Cook 35g porridge oats with 150ml skimmed milk, 100ml water and 1 rounded dspn raisins or sultanas. Add sweetener to taste.

12 ③ Beans & cheese jacket

Bake or microwave a 200g potato and fill with 4 rounded tbsp baked beans. Top with 15g grated half-fat cheddar and serve with No-Check salad.

up to 16 ⑯ Pizza

Serve any "healthy" vegetarian pizza up to a maximum of 400 calories and 16g fat (e.g. Marks & Spencer Count On Us Chargrilled Vegetable Pizza). Serve with No-Check salad, or have a bowl of No-Check soup for a starter.

Total meal Checks up to 36 ㉑

Don't forget to add Every Day Bonus foods and Essential Extras!

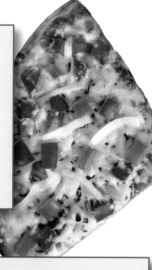

7 ⑤ Savoury toasted cheese

Mix 30g half-fat grated cheese with 1 tbsp fat-free natural fromage frais and 1 chopped spring onion. Grill one side of a medium slice of bread, spread mixture on other side and grill.

15 ⑦ Flame-grilled burgers

Grill 2 Linda McCartney Flame-grilled Burgers and serve on lightly toasted halves of 1 sesame seed bun with lettuce, tomato and 2 tsp relish.

10 ② Mushroom stroganoff

Soften a small chopped onion in pan sprayed with oil. Add 115g roughly chopped mushrooms, 1 crumbled vegetable Oxo cube, 1 tbsp tomato purée and pinch of thyme. Stir 1 minute. Add 100ml hot water and simmer 3-4 minutes. Remove pan from heat and stir in 2 rounded dspn fat-free natural fromage frais. Warm gently, stirring. Sprinkle with black pepper and chopped parsley. Serve with 60g dry weight boiled rice or tagliatelle and No-Check vegetables.

Total meal Checks 32 ⑭

Don't forget to add Every Day Bonus foods and Essential Extras!

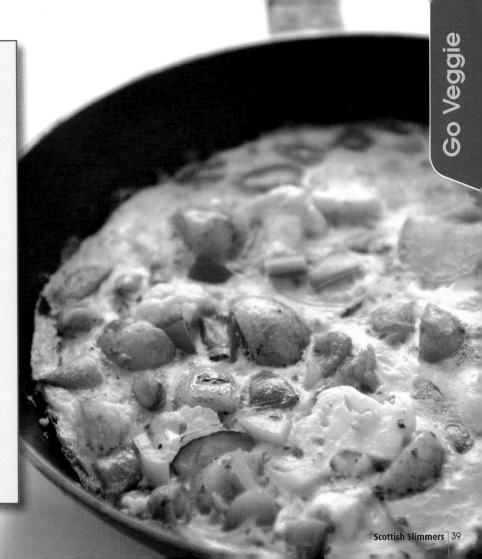

Sunday

7 6 Spanish tortilla

Take 150g cold, boiled potato and some cooked No-Check vegetables. Stir-fry in pan sprayed with oil until starting to brown. Beat 1 egg, pour over vegetables and cook gently until set underneath. Place under the grill to set top.

13 8 Cauliflower cheese

Boil and drain 350g cauliflower. Place 1 rounded dspn cornflour in a small non-stick saucepan, stir in 150ml skimmed milk and season to taste. Simmer gently, stirring continuously until thickened. Stir in ½ tsp mustard and 45g grated mature half-fat cheddar. Continue stirring until cheese has melted. Pour sauce over cauliflower and serve with 2 rounded tbsp peas and 1 medium slice bread.

16 13 Quorn Lemon & Black Pepper Escalope

Grill or ovenbake 1 Quorn Lemon & Black Pepper Escalope and serve with 200g new potatoes and No-Check vegetables.

Total meal Checks 36 27

Don't forget to add Every Day Bonus foods and Essential Extras!

Go Veggie Essential Extras

1 Tivall Frankfurter	3	5
1 Goodlife Organic Spicy Bean Quarter Pounder	8	7
1 Dalepak Vegetable Grill	6	9
2 slices Quorn Deli Chicken or Ham Style	1	0.5
1 Quorn Rasher	1.5	3

1 rounded tsp peanut butter	2	4
1 tbsp Baco's Bacon Flavour Soya Chips	1	1.5
115g Cauldron Foods Sweet Tomato, Lentil & Basil Pâté	7	8
70g jar Princes Roasted Red Pepper Pâté	4	4

1 sachet low-cal cup soup	2	1.5
30-35g Crispy Snack-a-Jacks	5	2
25g Jacob's Thai Bites	4	1
25g Twiglets Original	4	3
25g peanuts	6	12

1 Fox's Officially Low Fat Cookie	3.5	0.5
1 Jordans Frusli Bar	5	4
1 Quaker Chewee Bar	4	3
1 Mr Kipling Country Slice or Lemon Slice	5	5
1 mini hot cross bun	4	2

20g Green & Black choc bar	4	6
1 Panda Liquorice Bar	4	0
50g box Sula sugar-free sweets	5	0

1 level scoop ice cream	2	2
Green's Loony Tunes Sugar Free Jelly	No-Check	

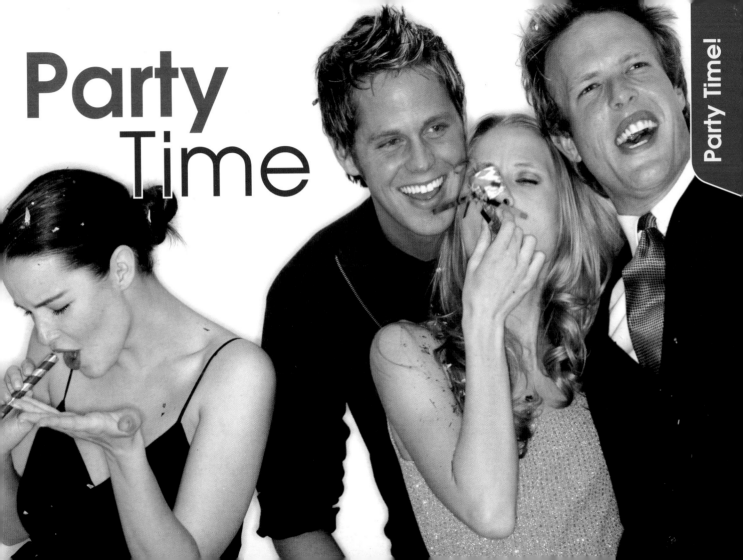

Party
Time

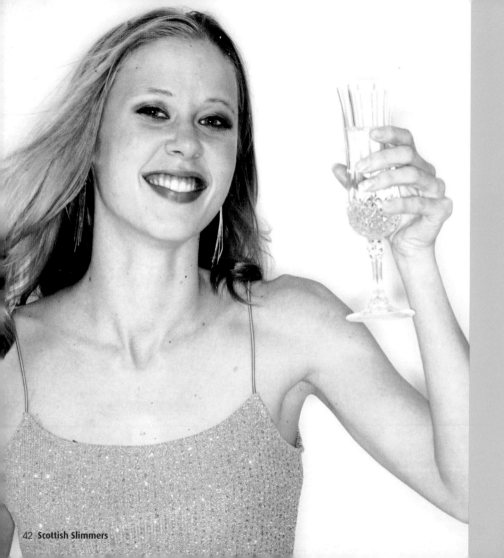

Losing weight doesn't mean you have to give up your social life – but if you want to party and still have a happy outcome on the scales at your weekly weigh-in, then there has to be some compensation somewhere!

Most members are familiar with the concept of saving a few Checks on less important days so that they can be a little more indulgent on days when they are socialising or perhaps just wish to have something a bit more special at weekends.

This plan is based on that concept but, as we all have different ideas on how we like to socialise, we have not been too prescriptive as to how you spend your saved Checks. Some people will want them for a couple of extra drinks on a Friday night out, others for a special Saturday evening meal out (or takeaway in), and others for a Sunday lunch with family and friends – or they could be needed for a midweek birthday treat.

Whenever and whatever you wish to spend them on, first you have to save some Checks, so in this plan we give ideas for four "stricter" days (which can be any days of the week you choose), and tell you how much you have left to spend on the other three days of the week (which can also be any days you choose).

The four "stricter" days are based on 35 Checks a day and include Every Day Bonus foods and Essential Extras. The amount you have to spend on the three "social days" will vary according to how many Checks a day you usually have. You can find the amount of Checks you have left to spend on your 3 "social days" in the chart following the "stricter" days.

> Note that the amounts given are the total to be spent over the three days – not the amount for each of the three days!

You can spend your "social days" Checks in any way you please, having more on one day than on the others, if you prefer.

Don't forget to add Every Day Bonus foods to your social days!

The four sample "stricter" days are only suitable if your usual daily Checks allowance for weight loss is up to 55

Checks a day. The stricter days would be too low if you normally have 60 or more Checks a day. However, if you do usually have 60 or more Checks a day, we give a separate chart suggesting how many Checks a day you could count on four "stricter" days of your own choice and the amount left for three "social" days. Every Day Bonus foods should be added to all days.

We've also included a reminder of some "social" Check values, but don't forget that the Social Scene section of our Check Book lists the Check and fat gram values of hundreds of alcoholic drinks, party foods, restaurant and takeaway meals – and now comes with a free mini "Going Out!" version you can pop into your handbag or jacket pocket.

So all you need now is to save, spend – and enjoy!

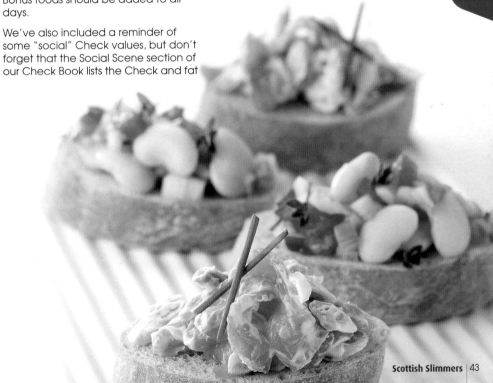

Stricter Day 1

EDB 150ml skimmed milk for use in drinks

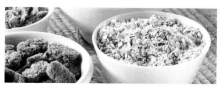

6 ① Cereal & milk

30g breakfast cereal with 150ml skimmed milk.

EDB 1 orange or 2 satsumas

9 ③ Chicken drumstick salad

Serve 2 skinless chicken drumsticks with a large No-Check salad and 1 medium slice bread.

EDB 1 apple or pear

14 ⑭ Favourite fish pie

Make sauce from 2 dspn Bisto Cheese Sauce Granules and 60ml boiling water. Mix in 85-100g can drained tuna and 2 dspn sweetcorn. Turn into ovenproof dish. Cover with sliced tomato and small pack crushed low-fat crisps mixed with 15g grated half-fat cheese. Bake in a moderate oven 25 minutes and serve with No-Check vegetables.

EDB 100g pot diet fromage frais

6 ④ 45g pack Kellogg's Nutri-grain Minis

Stricter Day 2

EDB 150ml skimmed milk for use in drinks

6 ⑤ Cheese on toast

Place 30g sliced half-fat cheese on 1 medium slice toast and grill until cheese melts.

EDB 2 small kiwi fruits or 3 plums

9 ① Pasta & bean soup

Cook together 45g pasta shapes, 3 tbsp canned kidney beans, 175g chopped No-Check vegetables, 200g canned tomatoes, 300ml stock and pinch of herbs. Bring to the boil, then simmer until tender.

EDB 1 peach or nectarine

14 ⑥ Sausage & mash

Grill 2 Wall's Lean Recipe or Quorn sausages. Boil 200g potato and mash with skimmed milk. Slice 1 onion and cook in spray oil. Make gravy from 1 dspn Oxo gravy granules. Mix with onions and pour over sausages. Serve with No-Check vegetables.

EDB 100g pot diet fromage frais

6 ④ 45g pack Kellogg's Nutri-grain Minis

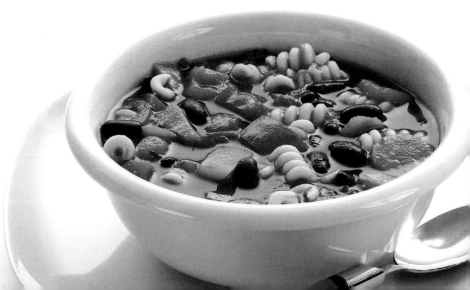

Stricter Day 3

EDB 150ml skimmed milk for use in drinks

6 7 Egg & toast

1 medium egg, boiled or poached. 1 medium slice wholemeal toast.

EDB 1 apple or pear

10 5 Prawn & pepper wrap

Cover 1 soft tortilla or wrap or chapatti with shredded lettuce, pepper strips, sliced spring onion, 60g prawns and 2 dspn sweet chilli sauce. Roll up and serve.

EDB 2 small kiwi fruits or 3 plums

13 3 Lemon & rosemary chicken

Place 1 skinless chicken breast on a square of foil. Season, top with 1 slice lemon and sprig of rosemary. Wrap into a parcel and bake in a moderate oven 25 minutes. Serve with 200g new potatoes, gravy made from 1 dspn Oxo granules and No-Check vegetables.

EDB 100g pot diet fromage frais

6 4 45g pack Kellogg's Nutri-grain Minis

Stricter Day 4

EDB 150ml skimmed milk for use in drinks

5 2 Rashers & toast

Grill tomatoes and 2 turkey rashers and serve with 1 medium slice wholemeal toast.

EDB 1 orange or 2 satsumas

10 4 Cottage cheese & pineapple jacket

Bake or microwave 200g potato in its jacket and fill with 2 heaped tbsp cottage cheese with pineapple. Serve with a large No-Check salad.

EDB 1 apple or pear

14 5 Spicy meatballs

Mix 85g turkey mince, half a small finely chopped onion, half slice bread, crumbed, pinch of cumin and chilli powder. Season. Form 6-8 balls and bake in a hot oven 15 minutes. Simmer 200g canned tomatoes with chopped pepper and garlic until thickened. Add meatballs and serve over 60g dry weight, boiled pasta.

EDB 100g pot diet fromage frais

6 4 45g pack Kellogg's Nutri-grain Minis

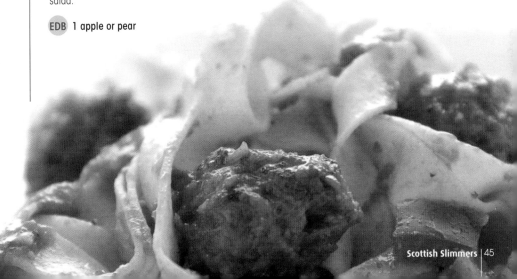

Having saved Checks on four days of the week, the tables below show how many Checks you can spend in total over the other three days of the week. The total amount can be spent in any way you please, spending more, or less, on some days than on others.

Up to 55 Checks per day

Usual daily Checks allowance	Total Checks for 3 "social" days
40	140
45	175
50	210
55	245

60 or more Checks per day

Usual daily Checks allowance	Daily Checks for 4 "stricter" days	Total Checks for 3 "social" days
60	45 per day	240
65	50 per day	255
70	55 per day	270
75	60 per day	285
80	65 per day	300

No-Check foods are ideal for filling the gap on "stricter" days.

No-Check Stuffed pepper

Halve 1 red pepper through the stalk and remove seeds. Fill with mushroom and tomato slices. Sprinkle with chopped garlic and pepper and spray with oil. Bake in pre-heated oven 190C/gas 5 approximately 30-45 minutes until starting to char at the edges.

Top tip

Keep a bowl of No-Check sugar-free jelly in the fridge to eat whenever you feel you need a little extra.

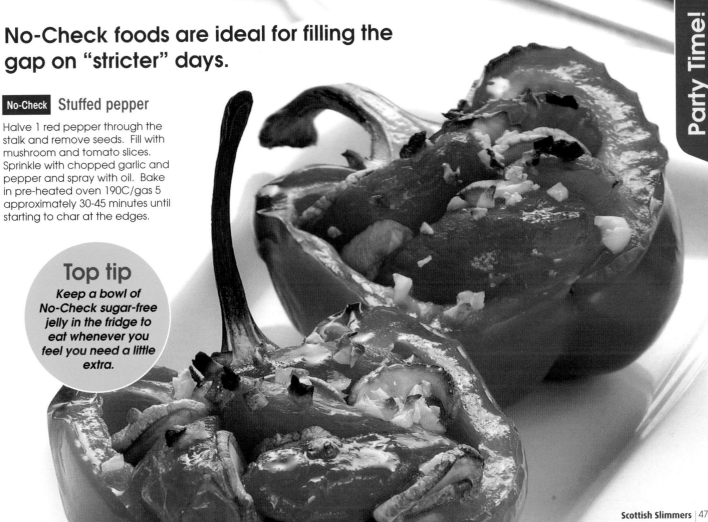

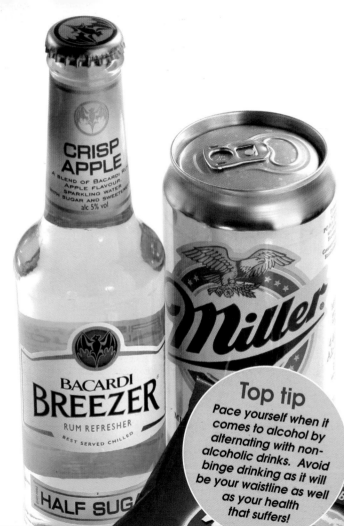

Party Time Essential Extras

125ml glass of wine	4	0
175ml glass of wine	5	0
125ml glass champagne	4	0
25ml shot of spirits	2	0
35ml shot of spirits	3	0
50ml Bailey's Irish Cream	7	8
50ml Tia Lusso	5	3
Half pint average strength beer, lager, cider	4	0
440-500ml bottle/can average strength beer, lager, cider	6	0
275ml Archers Vea	5	0
275ml Bacardi Breezer Half Sugar	5	0
275ml Red Square Reloaded	9	0
275ml Smirnoff Ice	7	0
275ml Vodka Source	7	0

Chicken Tikka Masala and Pilau Rice	50	53
Chicken Korma and Pilau Rice	55	63
Beef or Chicken Chow Mein	25	30
Beef or Chicken with Mushrooms or Peppers and Egg Fried or Special Fried Rice	35	32
Pizza Hut individual Chicken Highlight pizza	25	16
Pizza Hut individual Vegetarian Highlight pizza	23	15

Top tip
Pace yourself when it comes to alcohol by alternating with non-alcoholic drinks. Avoid binge drinking as it will be your waistline as well as your health that suffers!

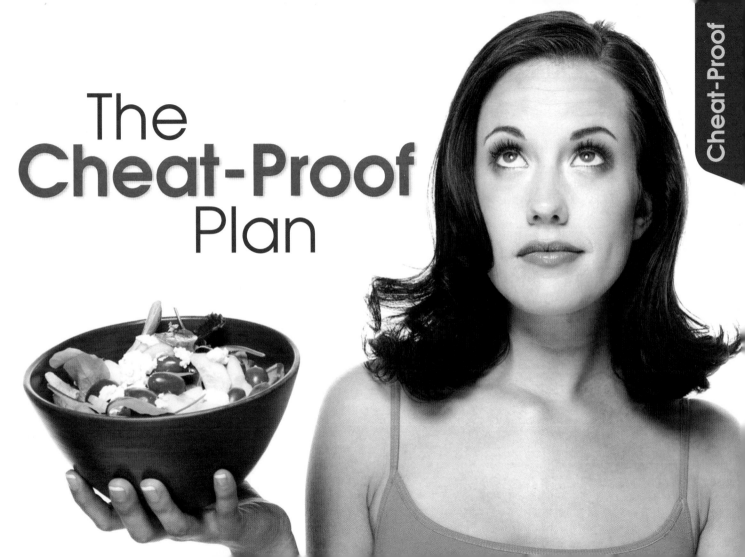

The
Cheat-Proof
Plan

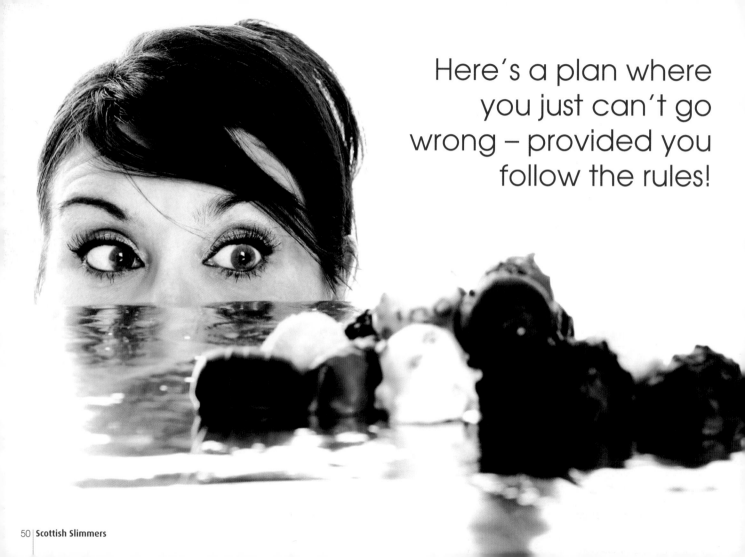

Here's a plan where you just can't go wrong – provided you follow the rules!

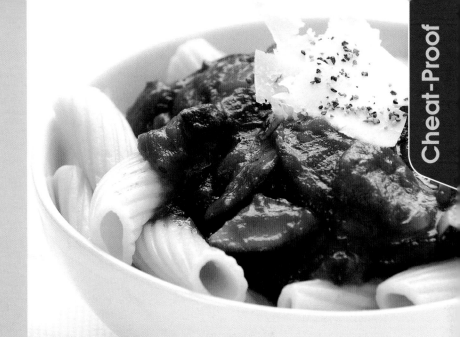

How to use it...

In the grid we've included everything you are allowed to eat during the week including all your Every Day Bonus foods. The only exception is that you may have additional No-Check veg if you wish.

This plan is particularly suitable for women on a daily Check allowance of 40-45, but if you are allowed more than this, there is just one small change you need to make. The plan allows for one small 400g loaf, but you can swap this for a large 800g loaf instead, all of which can be eaten during the week. You'll have about 6 extra (and larger) slices.

You can eat any food at any time. Cross items off the grid as you use them.

You are also allowed 14 "additions" during the week and you can make your choices from the list on page 56.

The other choice you have to make is what you want for your Essential Extras. Simply buy items from ONE box only.

Use the grid to make up your shopping list. If you add the weights of the same items together, you'll know how much you need. For example, 3 x 500ml cartons of skimmed milk and 200g/7 oz half-fat cheese. We've tried to use standard portion sizes to make shopping easy, but don't worry if a can size is a few grams more or less.

We've given some ideas for meals you could make using items from the grid but, if you prefer, you can be as creative as you like with the ingredients and have them any way you want.

JUST REMEMBER

when it's gone ... it's gone!

All you can eat...

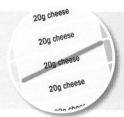

150ml milk	20g cheese	1 small yoghurt or fromage frais	1 chicken breast	1 chicken breast	150g lean chop or steak
150ml milk	20g cheese	1 small yoghurt or fromage frais	125g lean mince	125g lean mince	150g salmon or trout fillet
150ml milk	20g cheese	1 small yoghurt or fromage frais	2 thin slices ham	2 thin slices ham	2 thin slices ham
150ml milk	20g cheese	1 small yoghurt or fromage frais	2 thin slices ham	2 thin slices ham	1 ready meal up to 400 calories
150ml milk	20g cheese	1 egg	1 bread roll	2 small slices bread	2 small slices bread
150ml milk	20g cheese	1 egg	1 bread roll	2 small slices bread	2 small slices bread
150ml milk	20g cheese	1 egg	1 bread roll	2 small slices bread	Extra bread allowance
150ml milk	20g cheese	200g can baked beans	1 bread roll	2 small slices bread	30g cereal or 1 Oatso-Simple
150ml milk	20g cheese	100g can tuna or prawns	1 bread roll	2 small slices bread	30g cereal or 1 Oatso-Simple
150ml milk	20g cheese	100g can tuna or prawns	1 bread roll	2 small slices bread	30g cereal or 1 Oatso-Simple

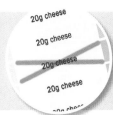

20g cheese

20g cheese

20g cheese

20g cheese

20g cheese

Complete the cross when you use the other half of the portion.

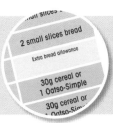

2 small slices bread

Extra bread allowance

30g cereal or 1 Oatso-Simple

30g cereal or 1 Oatso-Sim...

If using an 800g loaf instead of 400g (see instructions at beginning), you will have approximately 6 more (larger) slices if using a sliced loaf.

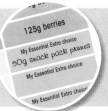

125g berries

My Essential Extra choice

50g snack pack prunes

My Essential Extra choice

My Essential Extra choice

Add in your Essential Extras – actual number of items may vary according to your choice.

60g dry, rice, pasta or noodles	250g stir-fry vegetables	2 carrots	1 apple	1 peach or 4 apricots	125g berries
60g dry, rice, pasta or noodles	250g stir-fry vegetables	2 carrots	1 apple	1 peach or 4 apricots	125g berries
60g dry, rice, pasta or noodles	1 red pepper	60g mushrooms	1 orange or 2 satsumas	2 kiwi fruit	125g berries
200g potato	Lettuce or salad leaves	60g mushrooms	1 orange or 2 satsumas	2 kiwi fruit	125g berries
200g potato	Lettuce or salad leaves	125g broccoli	1 addition	1 addition	My Essential Extra choice
200g new potatoes	Lettuce or salad leaves	125g broccoli	1 addition	1 addition	My Essential Extra choice
200g new potatoes	Lettuce or salad leaves	85g grapes or 2 pineapple rings	1 addition	1 addition	My Essential Extra choice
2 tomatoes	Lettuce or salad leaves	85g grapes or 2 pineapple rings	1 addition	1 addition	My Essential Extra choice
2 tomatoes	1 onion	2 plums	1 addition	1 addition	My Essential Extra choice
2 tomatoes	1 onion	2 plums	1 addition	1 addition	My Essential Extra choice
2 tomatoes	1 onion	2 plums	1 addition	1 addition	My Essential Extra choice

Meal Ideas

■ Egg & mushrooms on toast

Poach or dry-fry an egg and serve on toast with some grilled or dry-fried mushrooms.

■ Toast & ham

Top each slice of toast with a thin slice of ham. Use some spread from "additions" if you like.

■ Tasty toastie

Make a sandwich from 2 slices bread, some half-fat cheese, sliced tomato, black pepper and a few torn basil leaves. Spray lightly with oil and either grill or cook in a sandwich toaster

■ Broccoli & cheese soup with roll

Cook about 100 g/3-4 oz chopped fresh or frozen broccoli in 200 ml/ ⅓ pint stock until just tender. Stir in 150 ml/¼ pint skimmed milk, some black pepper and 40 g/1½ oz grated half-fat cheese. Serve with a bread roll.

■ Cheese & red pepper roll

Fill a roll with some lettuce, half-fat cheese and a couple of rings of crunchy red pepper.

■ Ham & egg salad

Prepare a salad of any No-Check veg. Add 1 hard-boiled egg and some ham. If you like, add some mayonnaise or salad cream from "additions" and serve with a slice of bread.

■ Tuna tops

Mix half the can of tuna with some chopped cucumber, tomato and spring onion. Mix with 2 dspn extra light mayonnaise or low-calorie salad cream. Split a roll in half and toast. Top each half with half the tuna mixture.

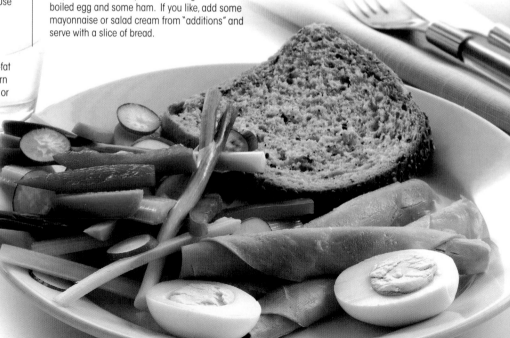

■ Chicken stir-fry

Cut 1 chicken breast into cubes and marinate 15 minutes in 1 dspn soy sauce and a tsp grated fresh ginger or a pinch of ground. Remove chicken and brown in pan sprayed with oil. Add fresh or frozen stir-fry veg and remaining marinade. Stir-fry until chicken is cooked through and vegetables are crisp-tender. Boil 60 g/2 oz portion rice or noodles and serve with chicken and vegetables.

■ Chicken with pan-fried potatoes

Sprinkle 1 chicken breast with herbs, wrap in foil and bake approx. 25 minutes in a moderate oven until juices run clear. Boil 200 g/7 oz new potatoes and cut into slices. Spray pan with oil and arrange slices over base. Allow to brown, turn over and brown other sides. Make gravy from 1 dsp Oxo or Bisto Best granules (1 "addition") and serve with No-Check vegetables.

■ Curried mince & vegetables

Soften 1 chopped onion and 1 crushed clove garlic in a saucepan sprayed with oil. Add 1 tbsp curry powder and stir 1 minute. Add 125 g/4½ oz mince and stir-fry until browned. Stir in 1 tbsp tomato purée, chopped carrot and broccoli and 200 ml/⅓ pint stock. Bring to a simmer, cover the pan and cook about 20 minutes, checking now and again, until the vegetables are tender. Boil 60 g/2 oz portion rice and serve with the curried mince.

■ Trout fillet with new potatoes

Microwave or grill 150 g/5 oz trout fillet and serve with wedges of lemon, 200 g/7 oz new potatoes and No-Check veg.

■ Honey & mustard pork with herby wedges

Grill a lean pork chop turning halfway through. About 5 minutes from end of cooking top with a mixture of 1 tsp honey (1 "addition") mixed with a little mustard. Bake or microwave a 200 g/7 oz potato, cut into wedges, spray with oil and sprinkle with mixed herbs. Brown under the grill or in a hot oven.

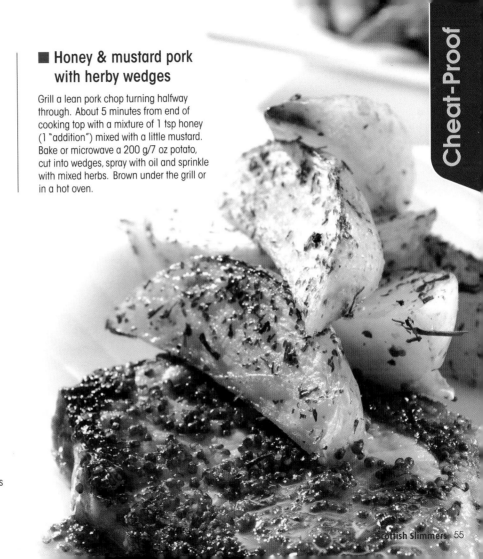

Storecupboard Check ✔

All the usual No-Check drinks and additions may be used.

Don't forget to check for items such as lemons, cans of tomatoes, your favourite herbs and spices, spray oil and sugar-free jelly.

You are also allowed 14 "servings" of any of the following "additions" during the week (choose the same or different as long as you don't have more than 14). Check you have those you are likely to use and add to your shopping list. The quantities given represent "1 serving".

1 tsp low-fat or olive oil spread
1 dspn low-calorie mayonnaise
2 dspn Hellman's Extra Light Mayonnaise
2 dspn low-calorie salad cream
1 dspn sweet chilli sauce
1 dspn pickles/chutney
1 dspn Oxo or Bisto Best gravy granules
5 olives
2 tsp reduced-sugar jam or marmalade
1 tsp honey
1 level tbsp cornflour
1 level tbsp custard powder

Cheat-Proof
Essential Extras

Choose ONE box only!

6 pack of Walkers French Fries
25cl can or bottle of wine or
2 x 275ml bottles Bacardi Breezers Half Sugar

150g pack Maryland Cookies or Fox's Chocolate Viennese or other pack of biscuits around 150g.
Or 140g pack of 7 Lunch Packs of Jammie Dodgers.

6-pack of low-fat/low-calorie cake slices
3 sachets Options or Highlights hot chocolate drinks

100g pack almonds or cashews or peanuts or mixed nuts, or pumpkin or sesame seeds
50g snack pack ready-to-eat apricots or prunes

4-pack Cadbury's Light Chocolate Mousse
3 x 150g pots Ambrosia Low Fat Rice Pudding or Custard

Choose your own combination of items up to 30 Checks/750 calories total. Either choose individual items or a multi-pack plus individual items to make up the calories. (It would be too tempting to buy several multi-packs with the intention of having only one or two items from each!)

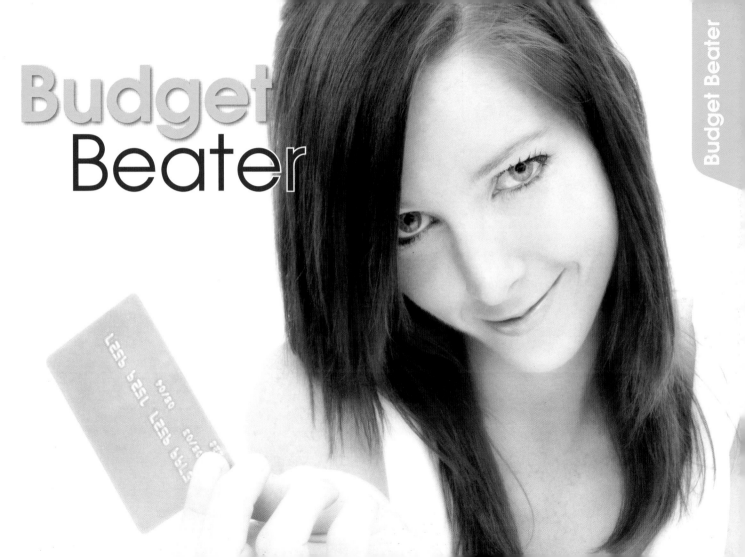

Budget
Beater

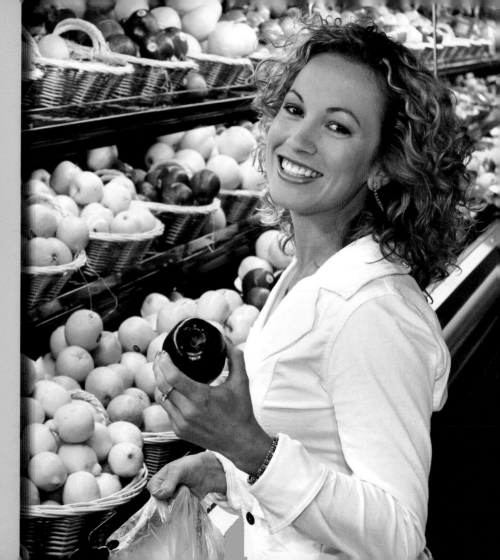

There's no need to spend a fortune in order to lose weight! Many inexpensive foods are packed with nutrition, and this plan shows how you can make the most of them.

In this plan we give examples of three meals a day and give the total number of Checks spent on meals. We've also included Every Day Bonus foods – so all you have to do is add your favourite Essential Extras up to your daily Check allowance.

Check in
at the check out!

Shop less frequently – you'll save money and be less tempted to buy goodies that are way above your Check allowance.

Batch cooking can save fuel costs, but freeze in individual portions so you're less tempted to finish it all up.

Plan ahead and stick with your shopping list.

Take care with multi-buys and "bogof" offers – if you're not feeding an army, you could end up throwing half of it away, or eating much more than you should.

Think about portion sizes and avoid the temptation to pay a little extra and "go large". It may seem like a bargain at the time, but not if it prevents you reaching Target Weight.

Freeze sliced loaves and take out a few slices at a time.

Some supermarket "economy" ranges include very reasonably priced healthy foods. Look out for skimmed milk, unsweetened juices, porridge, muesli, bran flakes, carrots, onions, peppers, skinless chicken breasts, quick-fry steaks, wholemeal bread, canned tomatoes, canned kidney beans and baked beans.

Canned oily fish such as sardines or pilchards in tomato sauce provide an inexpensive way to get your weekly dose of heart-healthy omega 3s.

Save money by growing a few herbs in your garden or on your kitchen windowsill. Freshly cut herbs can add lots of vitamin C to a meal. You can also freeze some of the excess for winter months when they don't grow as well.

There's no waste with frozen vegetables, and they often have more vitamins than fresh ones that have travelled half way round the world or have been on the shelf for a long time.

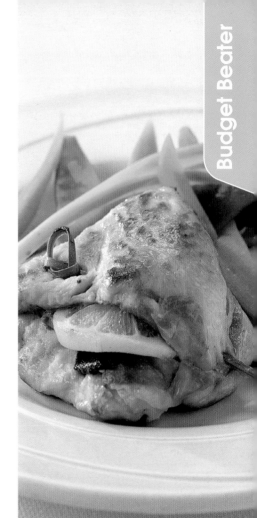

Monday

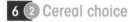

EDB 150ml skimmed milk for use in drinks

EDB 200ml unsweetened orange juice

6 2 Cereal choice

30g of your favourite wholegrain cereal with 150ml skimmed milk.

12 7 Cheese salad sandwich & apple

Spread 2 medium slices wholemeal bread with 1 tsp low-fat spread and fill with 30g half-fat cheese, lettuce and tomato. 1 apple or pear.

16 11 Corned beef & cabbage stir-fry

Boil and drain 60g Chinese noodles. Stir-fry 1 sliced onion, some chopped/shredded fresh or frozen cabbage and some frozen mixed peppers in a pan sprayed with oil. Add 100g cubed lean corned beef and warm through. Season with a little soy sauce and serve with noodles.

EDB 125g pot diet yoghurt

Checks spent on meals	34

Don't forget to add your Essential Extras!

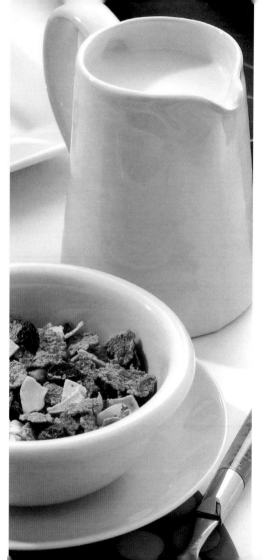

Tuesday

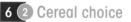

EDB 150ml skimmed milk for use in drinks

EDB 200ml unsweetened orange juice

6 2 Cereal choice

30g of your favourite wholegrain cereal with 150ml skimmed milk.

12 11 Corned beef salad

Prepare a salad of No-Check vegetables. Add 50g lean corned beef, 1 tsp pickles or relish and serve with 2 medium slices wholemeal bread with 1 tsp low-fat spread.

16 6 Fish in sauce with mash & peas

Boil or microwave 1 individual portion Young's Cod Steak in Butter or Parsley Sauce. Boil and mash 200g potatoes. Serve with 3 rounded tbsp peas and other No-Check vegetables. Follow with 1 pear.

EDB 125g pot diet yoghurt

Checks spent on meals	34

Don't forget to add your Essential Extras!

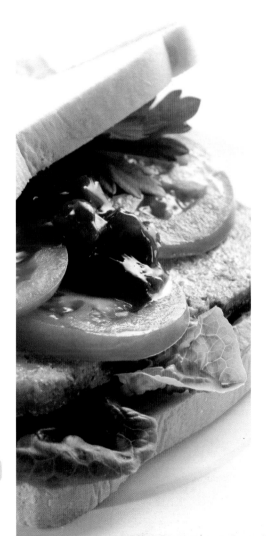
Wednesday

EDB 150ml skimmed milk for use in drinks

EDB 200ml unsweetened orange juice

6 5 Cheese on toast

Place 30g sliced half-fat cheese on 1 medium slice wholemeal toast and grill until melted. Serve with grilled tomato.

10 11 Egg salad sandwich

Fill 2 medium slices wholemeal bread with lettuce, 1 sliced hard-boiled medium egg and 1 dspn low-calorie mayonnaise or salad cream.

16 14 Pork shoulder chop

Trim excess fat from 200g on the bone pork shoulder chop. Cook covered in a low oven until very tender. Serve with 200g potatoes, gravy made from 1 dspn Oxo gravy granules, cabbage and carrots or other No-Check vegetables.

EDB 125g pot diet yoghurt

Checks spent on meals 32 30

Don't forget to add your Essential Extras!

Thursday

EDB 150ml skimmed milk for use in drinks

EDB 200ml unsweetened orange juice

6 2 Cereal choice

30g of your favourite wholegrain cereal with 150ml skimmed milk.

12 11 Corned beef sandwich

Spread 2 medium slices wholemeal bread with 1 tsp low-fat spread and fill with lettuce, 50g lean corned beef and 1 tsp pickles or relish.

17 22 Cheese & pepper omelette with chips

Stir-fry a good handful of frozen mixed peppers in pan sprayed with oil. Stir in 2 beaten medium eggs and cook gently until set underneath. Sprinkle with 30g grated half-fat cheese and place under the grill to melt cheese and set top. Serve with 100g frozen weight, low-fat oven chips and 2 tbsp peas.

EDB 125g pot diet yoghurt

Checks spent on meals 35 35

Don't forget to add your Essential Extras!

Friday

EDB 150ml skimmed milk for use in drinks

EDB 200ml unsweetened orange juice

6 2 Cereal choice

30g of your favourite wholegrain cereal with 150ml skimmed milk.

11 7 Tuna salad

Prepare a large salad of No-Check vegetables and add 85-100g can drained tuna in brine, 1 dspn low-calorie mayonnaise or salad cream and serve with 2 medium slices wholemeal bread and 1 tsp low-fat spread.

19 6 Baked bean lasagne

Cook chopped onion and mushrooms in spray oil. Add 200g baked beans, 1 chopped tomato, garlic powder and mixed herbs. Layer mixture between 3 lasagne sheets in an ovenproof dish. Make sauce from 1 dspn cornflour, 150ml skimmed milk, 30g grated half-fat cheese, ½ tsp mustard. Heat gently, stirring until thickened. Pour over lasagne and bake 200C/gas 6 approximately 30 minutes.

EDB (3g fat) 20g half-fat cheddar (may be added to lasagne sauce if preferred).

Checks spent on meals 36 18

Don't forget to add your Essential Extras!

Saturday

EDB 150ml skimmed milk for use in drinks

8 8 Scrambled egg & beans

Scramble 1 medium egg in a non-stick pan or microwave. Reserve 2 tbsp baked beans from 200g (for today's main meal) and serve remainder with egg.

12 14 Pilchards on toast

Warm 155g can pilchards in tomato sauce and serve with 1 medium slice wholemeal toast.

16 8 Chilli con carne

Brown 85g lean mince with chopped onion and garlic. Drain any surplus fat. Add 200g canned tomatoes, 1 tbsp tomato purée, 2 tbsp baked beans, frozen sliced peppers, cumin and chilli powder to taste. Simmer until vegetables are tender. Season to taste. Serve with 60g dry weight boiled rice.

EDB 1 medium banana

EDB Vanilla milk
Heat 200ml skimmed milk and flavour with a few drops of vanilla essence and sweetener to taste.

Checks spent on meals 36 30

Don't forget to add your Essential Extras!

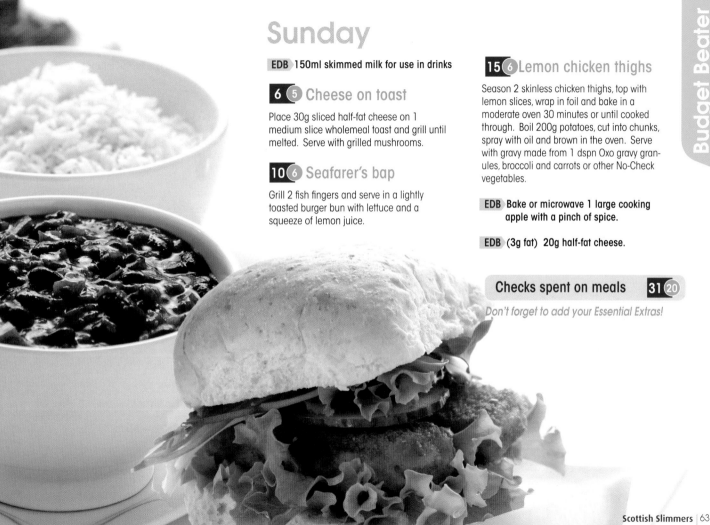

Sunday

EDB 150ml skimmed milk for use in drinks

6 5 Cheese on toast

Place 30g sliced half-fat cheese on 1 medium slice wholemeal toast and grill until melted. Serve with grilled mushrooms.

10 6 Seafarer's bap

Grill 2 fish fingers and serve in a lightly toasted burger bun with lettuce and a squeeze of lemon juice.

15 6 Lemon chicken thighs

Season 2 skinless chicken thighs, top with lemon slices, wrap in foil and bake in a moderate oven 30 minutes or until cooked through. Boil 200g potatoes, cut into chunks, spray with oil and brown in the oven. Serve with gravy made from 1 dspn Oxo gravy granules, broccoli and carrots or other No-Check vegetables.

EDB Bake or microwave 1 large cooking apple with a pinch of spice.

EDB (3g fat) 20g half-fat cheese.

Checks spent on meals 31 20

Don't forget to add your Essential Extras!

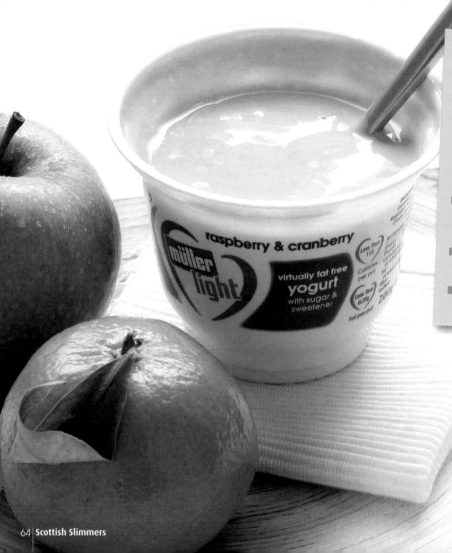

Shopping tips

- **2 x 1 ltr cartons skimmed milk is sufficient for all your needs.**

- 1 ltr carton unsweetened orange juice for 5 x 200ml servings.

- **Choose your favourite 4 x 125g pack of diet yoghurts.**

- 200g can of corned beef will make main meal on Monday and quick meals on Tuesday and Thursday.

- **190g half-fat cheese is required. If you have to buy more, use as Essential Extras.**

- Useful frozen vegetables would be cabbage, carrots, sliced mixed peppers, broccoli, peas.

Essential Extras

1 Ryvita Original or Dark Rye	1	0
1 medium slice wholemeal bread/toast	3	1
30g half-fat cheddar	3	5
2 McVitie's Light Hob Nobs	5	5
2-finger Kit Kat	4	6
23g pack Walker's Potato Heads	4	5
1 level scoop ice cream	2	2

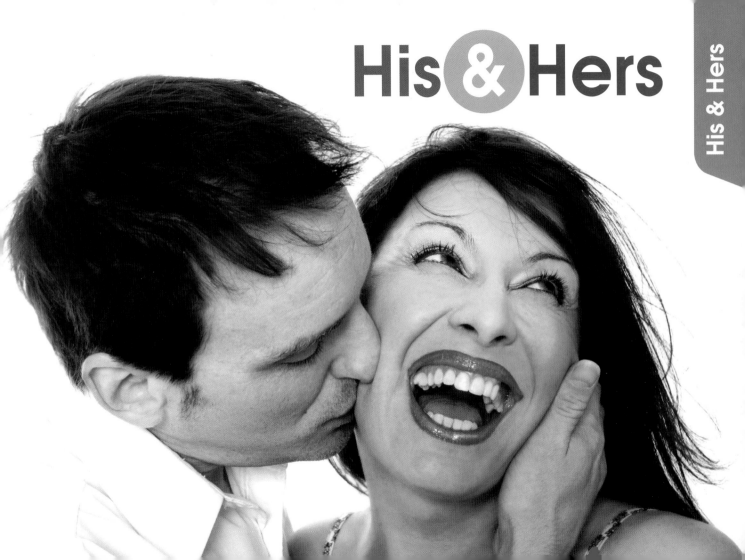

His&Hers

If your partner wants to
lose weight, or if you feel
that they should eat more
healthily, follow this 7-day
His 'n' Hers Plan which makes
cooking – and slimming –
for two, simple!

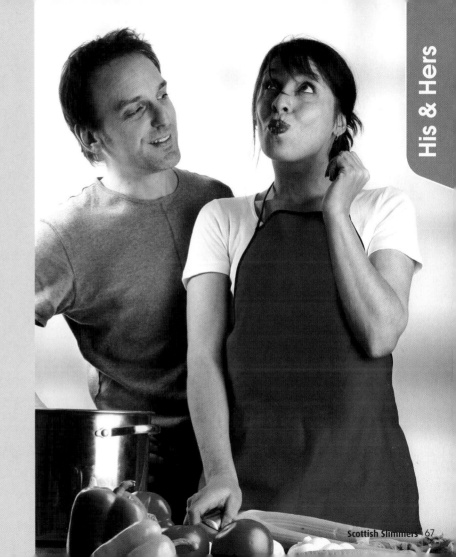

If your partner doesn't need to lose weight, you can simply add extra portions of bread, potatoes, pasta, rice etc. to his meals, or have additional snacks.

(If overweight, most men will lose on around 60-70 Checks a day. If he doesn't need to lose weight, around 70-80 Checks a day would be suitable for most men trying to maintain average weight).

Usual Every Day Bonus foods (milk/yoghurt, fruit, vegetables, No-Check drinks and additions) should be added by both partners to the meals listed.

At the end of each day we give the total amount of Checks and fat grams spent by each person on meals. Each partner can add their preferred Essential Extras, up to their daily Checks allowance.

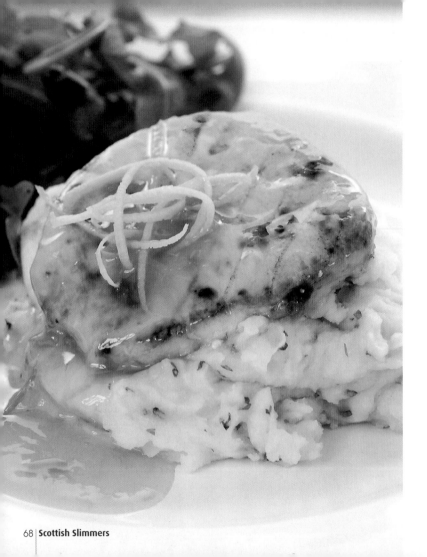

Monday

Cereal choice

HERS 8 (4) **HIS 10** (6)

45g any cereal, muesli or porridge with 150ml skimmed milk extra to Every Day Bonus allowance.

HIS Increase cereal to 60g.

Salmon salad or sandwich

HERS 10 (9) **HIS 14** (12)

Share a 200g can of pink salmon. Serve with lots of No-Check salad, 1 medium slice bread and 1 tsp low-fat spread.

HIS Add 1 additional slice bread and 1 tsp low-fat spread, so his could be served as a sandwich, if preferred.

Marmalade pork with parsley mash

HERS 16 (7) **HIS 18** (7)

Grill 2 well-trimmed, medium pork loin chops. Soften a small, sliced onion in spray oil. Mix 1 tsp cornflour with 1 tbsp water and 200ml unsweetened orange juice. Stir juice into onions together with 1 dspn grated orange zest, ½ Knorr chicken cube and 1 tbsp reduced-sugar marmalade. Simmer until thickened. Boil and mash 450g potatoes with skimmed milk and 2 tbsp chopped parsley. Serve with No-Check vegetables.

HIS He gets a bit more than half the mash!

Checks spent on meals

HERS 34 (20) **HIS 42** (25)

Tuesday

Egg & toast

HERS 7 (9) **HIS** 11 (12)

1 medium egg, boiled or poached, served with 1 medium slice toast and 1 tsp low-fat spread.

HIS ▸ Add 1 additional slice toast and spread.

Cheese salad sandwich

HERS 11 (10) **HIS** 15 (13)

Spread 2 medium slices bread with low-fat spread and fill with 30g half-fat cheese and lots of No-Check salad.

HIS ▸ Add 1 additional slice bread and spread and make into a double-decker.

Bacon & peppers pasta

HERS 18 (8) **HIS** 18 (8)

Boil 175g pasta until al dente. Cook sliced onion and peppers in pan sprayed with oil. Add 60g lean chopped back bacon and brown. Stir in 320g jar Dolmio Light pasta sauce. Heat through and serve over drained pasta.

HIS ▸ Share equally!

Checks spent on meals

HERS 36 (27) **HIS** 44 (33)

Wednesday

Cereal choice

HERS 8 (4) **HIS** 10 (6)

45g any cereal, muesli or porridge with 150ml skimmed milk extra to Every Day Bonus allowance.

HIS ▸ Increase cereal to 60g.

Tuna mayo sandwich or jacket

HERS 11 (7) **HIS** 18 (13)

Drain and mix together 100g plus 200g can tuna in water or brine. Add chopped tomato, cucumber and spring onion and 3 tbsp low-calorie mayonnaise.

HERS ▸ Take one-third of the mixture and use to fill either 2 medium slices bread or a 200g potato, microwaved or baked. Serve with No-Check salad.

HIS ▸ As Hers, but using two-thirds of the mixture and either 3 medium slices bread or a 300g potato.

Sausage & mash

HERS 13 (7) **HIS** 18 (10)

Grill 8 Wall's Lean Recipe Sausages. Serve 3 to Him and 2 to Her. Reserve remaining 3 for tomorrow's lunch. Boil 450g potatoes and mash with a little skimmed milk and mustard to taste (optional). Serve a bit more than one-third to Her and the rest to Him. Make gravy from 2 dspn Oxo granules and share. Serve with No-Check vegetables.

Checks spent on meals

HERS 32 (18) **HIS** 46 (29)

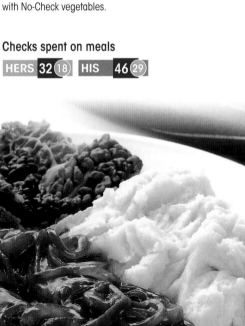

Thursday

Egg & toast

HERS 7 **HIS** 11

1 medium egg, boiled or poached, served with 1 medium slice toast and 1 tsp low-fat spread.

HIS Add 1 additional slice toast and spread.

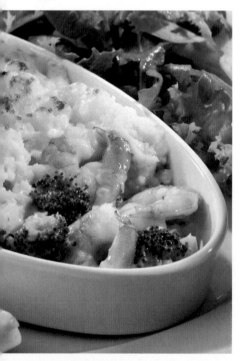

Sausage sarnie

HERS 11 **HIS** 14

Spread 2 medium slices bread with 1 tsp low-fat spread and mustard to taste. Slice 1 cooked sausage, reserved from yesterday and use to fill sandwich together with sliced tomatoes.

HIS As Hers, using 2 remaining sausages.

Fish & prawn pie

HERS 16 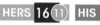 **HIS** 16

Boil 450g potatoes. Drain and mash with a little skimmed milk. Boil or microwave 175g broccoli, drain and chop. Boil or microwave 2 x 170g packs Birds Eye Fish in Butter Sauce according to pack instructions. In a heatproof dish, mix chopped broccoli with 60g prawns and fish in sauce. Top with mashed potato and brown under the grill. Share equally and serve with green beans or other No-Check vegetables.

Checks spent on meals

HERS 34 **HIS** 41

Friday

Cereal choice

HERS 8 **HIS** 10

45g any cereal, muesli or porridge with 150ml skimmed milk extra to Every Day Bonus allowance.

HIS Increase cereal to 60g.

Corned beef salad

HERS 12 **HIS** 16

Share a small 200g can of corned beef. Serve with lots of No-Check salad and 1 medium slice bread.

HIS Add 1 additional slice bread and 1 tsp low-fat spread so His could be served as a sandwich, if preferred.

Chicken & cashew nuts with egg fried rice

HERS 20 **HIS** 20

Cut 2 skinless chicken breasts into strips. Mix 1 tsp cornflour with 1 tsp soy sauce and 1 tsp sherry and coat the chicken. Crush 1 clove garlic, grate a small knob of ginger, slice 2 spring onions and cut 1 carrot into strips. Spray pan with oil and stir-fry vegetables 2 minutes. Add the coated chicken and cook 2-3 minutes more. Add 30g cashew nuts and 2 tbsp hoisin sauce. Stir-fry until chicken is cooked through. Boil 60g rice. Chop and stir-fry in spray oil, 2 spring onions, handful of peppers, chopped clove garlic and 1 dspn grated fresh ginger. Remove from pan. Re-spray and add 1 beaten egg, breaking it up as it cooks. Add vegetables, cooked rice, 2 tbsp peas and soy sauce to taste. Heat through. Divide chicken and rice equally.

Checks spent on meals

HERS 40 **HIS** 46

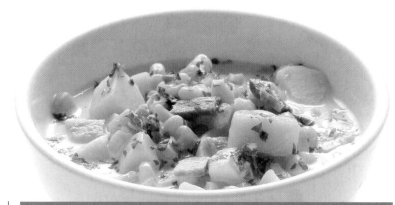

Saturday

Cheese on toast

HERS 6 **HIS** 12

30g half-fat cheese melted on 1 medium slice toast, served with grilled tomatoes.

HIS Increase to 60g half-fat cheese and 2 slices toast.

Potato, sweetcorn & ham chowder

HERS 11 **HIS** 11

Roughly chop 10 canned new potatoes and place in a saucepan together with 4 tbsp sweetcorn kernels, 60g shredded lean ham and 400ml skimmed milk. Warm through stirring frequently. Season to taste and sprinkle with chopped parsley. Share equally.

Steak & chips

HERS 16 **HIS** 20

Ovenbake 300g frozen weight McCain's Home Fries. Share equally. Season and grill Her 150g and His 225g lean rump steak. Serve with green beans or broccoli, grilled mushrooms and tomatoes or other No-Check vegetables or salad.

Checks spent on meals

HERS 33 **HIS** 43

Sunday

Rise & shine

HERS 8 **HIS** 9

Share a pink grapefruit and sprinkle with sweetener if required. Scramble 2 medium eggs in a non-stick pan. Serve half to each on 1 medium slice toast each. Grill 3 turkey rashers and some tomatoes. Serve 1 rasher to Her and 2 to Him.

Prawn & pepper wrap

HERS 10 **HIS** 20

Cover 1 soft tortilla or wrap or chapatti with shredded lettuce, pepper strips, sliced spring onions, 60g prawns and 2 dspn sweet chill sauce. Roll up and serve.

HIS Make 2 wraps as above.

Roast Dinner

HERS 17 **HIS** 23

Roast your favourite lean meat or poultry. Cut a 200g potato into 3 chunks and a 275g potato into 4 chunks. Boil, drain then spray with oil and roast in a hot oven. Make gravy from 2 dspn Oxo gravy granules and 150ml boiling water.

HERS Serve 2 good slices lean meat, half the gravy, 3 chunks potato and No-Check vegetables.

HIS Serve 3 good slices lean meat, half the gravy, 4 chunks potato and No-Check vegetables.

Checks spent on meals

HERS 35 **HIS** 52

His&Hers Essential Extras

1 medium slice bread	3	1
50g bread roll	5	2
60g small currant bun	6	3
30g dry weight, pasta or rice	4	0.5
1 Paterson's Oatcake	2	2
1 Ryvita Original or Dark Rye	1	0
30g brie	4	8
30g half-fat cheddar	3	4

1 level scoop plain ice cream	2	2
Danone Goodies Strawberry Trifle	6	2
140g M&S COU Bread & Butter Pudding	6	3
145g Muller Amoré Continental Mousse	8	6
100g pot crème caramel	4	1
1 Mr Kipling Apple Pie	9	9

2 McVitie's Light Hob Nobs	5	5
40g Fox's Officially Low Fat Minis	6	1
1 Quaker Dipps	5	5
1 Alpen Light Bar	3	1
1 Tunnocks Teacake	4	4

25g Jacob's Thai Bites	4	1
33g Walkers Doritos	7	9
2-finger Kit Kat	4	6
68g Yorkie	15	22

125ml glass wine	4	0
440ml can 3-5% ABV beer or lager	6	0

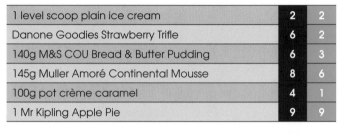

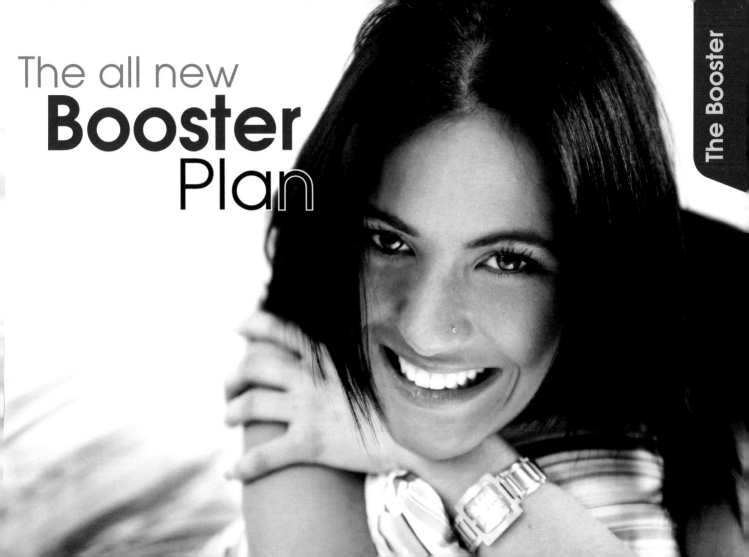

The all new
Booster
Plan

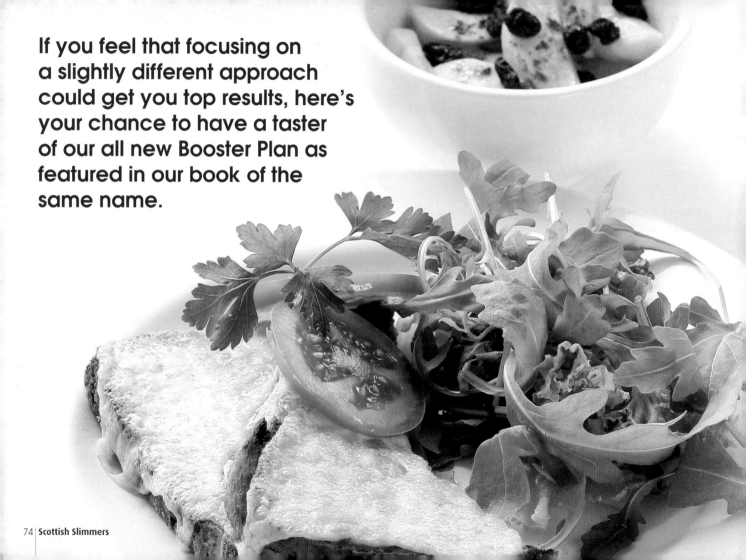

If you feel that focusing on a slightly different approach could get you top results, here's your chance to have a taster of our all new Booster Plan as featured in our book of the same name.

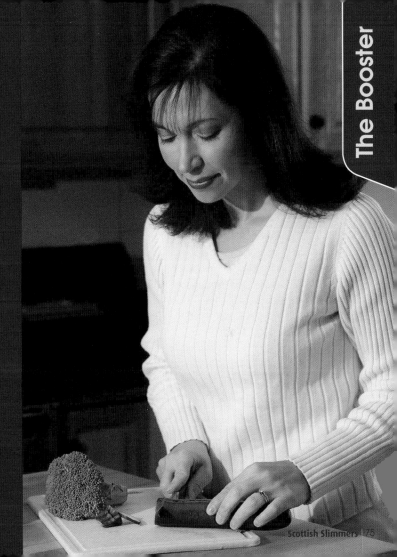

Whilst retaining all our usual Positive Eating features such as Every Day Bonus foods and using Checks, there is one major difference.

On this Booster Plan, there are many foods which don't need to be counted at all. These include lean meat, fish, eggs, Quorn, low-fat dairy produce and pulses, so there is less weighing to do, and more that can be eaten freely according to your appetite. Of course there has to be a trade-off – and that is that all women have just 20 Checks a day to spend on other foods, but with so many "No-Need-To-Count" foods, you'll find these 20 Checks go a lot further! All men have 30 Checks a day to spend.

Another difference is that, you don't need to "save" Checks for the weekend or a special treat as, in addition to your daily Checks allowance, you also have a Special Weekly Allowance of an extra 20 Checks which can be spent at any time during the week, or not at all if you don't need them.

Of course, everything is explained in detail in the book, but whilst most Essential Extras are counted in exactly the same way as on other Positive Eating Plans, a few items are counted differently if they are a combination of No-Need-To-Count foods and foods that should be counted. A good example is a "healthy" ready meal where the meat or fish doesn't need to be counted but the potatoes, rice or pasta does. To keep things simple, you just count half the normal Checks!

The following example is based on 20 "Checks to count" and includes Every Day Bonus foods, so men wishing to use this plan should add another 10 Checks.

If you enjoy using this plan, our All New Booster Plan – Lose a Stone in Six Weeks can be purchased in class or from our order-line.

Monday ●●●

 Checks to count 0 Skimmed milk for use in drinks

 Checks to count 4 ## Special K

30g Special K with Red or Purple Berries with skimmed milk.

EDB 1 apple or pear

 Checks to count 7 ## Chicken salad sandwich

Spread 1 tsp low-fat spread on 2 medium slices wholemeal bread and fill with cooked chicken and No-Check salad.

EDB 1 orange

 Checks to count 6 ## Spaghetti bolognese

Brown a medium portion of lean mince with chopped onion and garlic. Add 200g canned tomatoes, half a small stock cube, pinch of herbs, chopped mushrooms and peppers. Simmer until sauce thickens. Serve with 45g dry weight, boiled pasta and top with some grated half-fat cheese.

EDB 200g pot Mullerlight yoghurt

Checks to count 3 1 Fox's Officially Low Fat or M&S Count On Us cereal bar

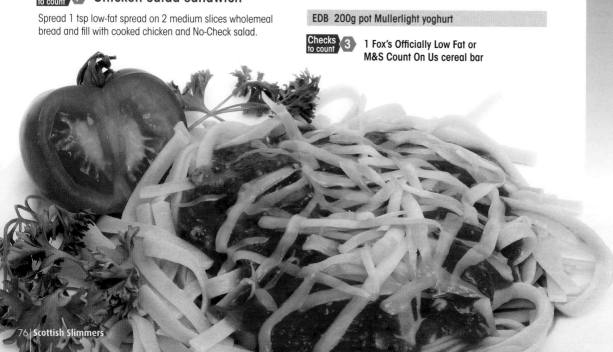

Tuesday ●●●

 0 Skimmed milk for use in drinks

 3 ## Scrambled egg on toast

Scramble 1 or 2 eggs with a little skimmed milk and serve on 1 medium slice wholemeal toast.

EDB 2 small kiwi fruits

 5 ## Tuna salad

Prepare a large No-Check salad. Add some drained tuna in brine, 1 dspn low-calorie mayonnaise, 1 medium slice wholemeal bread and 1 tsp low-fat spread.

EDB 1 peach or nectarine

 7 ## Ham & cheese chicken

Wrap 1 slice thin ham around 15g half-fat cheddar. Slit a pocket in a skinless chicken breast and push in ham-wrapped cheese. Secure with a cocktail stick. Cook in pan sprayed with oil. Serve with 200g potatoes boiled and mashed with skimmed milk, gravy made from 1 dspn Oxo gravy granules and No-Check vegetables.

EDB 200g pot Mullerlight yoghurt

 5 26g pack Scottish Slimmers Mini Cookies.

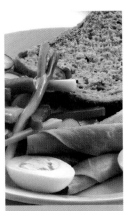

Wednesday ●●●

 0 Skimmed milk for use in drinks

 4 ## Ryvita & soft cheese

Spread light or extra light soft cheese on 4 Ryvita Original or Dark Rye crispbreads.

EDB 1 small kiwi fruit

5 ## Ham & egg salad

Prepare a large No-Check salad. Add some lean ham, 1 hard-boiled egg and 1 dspn low-calorie mayonnaise. 1 medium slice wholemeal bread with 1 tsp low-fat spread.

EDB 1 small kiwi fruit

8 ## Corned beef hash

Sauté 1 chopped onion in spray oil. Add 275g cooked potato, cooked carrot, turnip/swede or other No-Check vegetables. Add a medium portion of cubed corned beef, mash together if preferred. Brown under the grill. Serve with No-Check salad or grilled tomatoes.

EDB 1 apple or pear

EDB 40g half-fat cheese

 3 1 Fox's Officially Low Fat or M&S COU cereal bar

Thursday ●●●

 Checks to count 0 Skimmed milk for use in drinks

 Checks to count 4 Special K

30g Special K with skimmed milk.

EDB 85g grapes

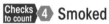 **Checks to count 4** Smoked mackerel salad

Prepare a large No-Check salad. Add some smoked mackerel fillets (may be topped with black pepper or mustard seeds). Serve with 1 medium slice bread with 1 tsp low-fat spread.

EDB 200g pot Mullerlight yoghurt

 Checks to count 7 Grilled lamb chops

Grill some well-trimmed lamb chops and serve with 200g new potatoes, gravy made from 1 dspn Oxo gravy granules, peas and other No-Check vegetables

EDB Microwave 3 halved plums with a pinch of cinnamon.

 Checks to count 5 26g pack Scottish Slimmers Mini Cookies

Friday ●●●

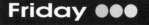

 Checks to count 0 Skimmed milk for use in drinks

 Checks to count 3 Turkey rashers & toast

Grill some turkey rashers and mushrooms and serve with 1 medium slice wholemeal toast.

EDB 85g grapes

 Checks to count 6 Ryvita & soft cheese

Spread light or extra light soft cheese on 6 Ryvita Original or Dark Rye crispbreads. Serve with cherry tomatoes, cucumber or other No-Check salad.

EDB 3 plums

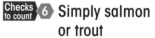 **Checks to count 6** Simply salmon or trout

Grill, steam or microwave salmon or trout fillet(s) and serve with 200g new potatoes, peas and other No-Check vegetables.

EDB 200g pot Mullerlight yoghurt

 Checks to count 5 26g pack Scottish Slimmers Mini Cookies.

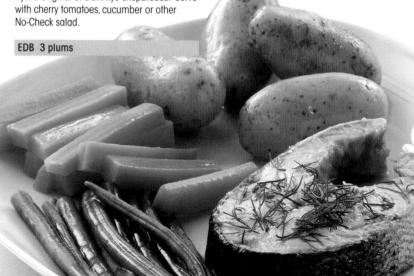

Saturday ●●●

 Checks to count 0 Skimmed milk for use in drinks

 Checks to count 3 Cheese on toast

Cover 1 medium slice wholemeal toast with grated half-fat cheese and grill until melted. Serve with grilled tomatoes.

> **EDB** Blitz 1 peeled nectarine or peach (or 2 drained, canned-in-juice peach halves) with about 200ml skimmed milk. Add sweetener to taste.

 Checks to count 0 Healthy burger & beans

Serve 1 grilled low-fat quarterpounder (e.g. Tesco Healthy Living, Sainsbury's Be Good To Yourself, Iceland Good Choice) with some baked beans.

 Checks to count 9 Quick tandoori chicken

Cut a skinless chicken breast into cubes and cook in a non-stick pan with 1 dspn Patak's Tandoori Curry Paste. Boil 50g rice with 4 cardomom pods and/or cloves, 1 bay leaf and ½ tsp turmeric. Serve with No-Check salad and 1 rounded tsp mango chutney.

> **EDB** A bowl of strawberries

 Checks to count 3 55g pot Cadbury's Light Chocolate Mousse

 Checks to count 5 26g pack Scottish Slimmers Mini Cookies.

Sunday ●●●

 Checks to count 0 Skimmed milk for use in drinks

 Checks to count 0 Rashers, egg & beans

Grill turkey rasher(s), poach or dry-fry an egg(s) and serve with baked beans.

 Checks to count 6 Prawn salad wrap

Cover 1 Discovery Foods Soft Flour Tortilla or Old El Paso Salsa Tortilla with shredded lettuce, a medium portion of prawns and 1 dspn low-calorie mayonnaise. Roll up and serve with additional No-Check salad.

 Checks to count 8 Roast pork

Serve some lean roast pork with gravy made from 1 dspn Oxo gravy granules. Peel and par-boil 200g potatoes, cut into chunks, spray with oil and roast in a hot oven. Serve with 1 tbsp apple sauce and No-Check vegetables.

> **EDB** 1 medium banana

Checks to count 3 55g pot Cadbury's Light Chocolate Mousse

> **EDB** 40g half-fat cheese

 Checks to count 3 3 Ryvita Original or Dark Rye and some cherry tomatoes

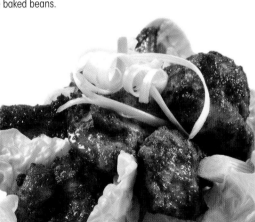

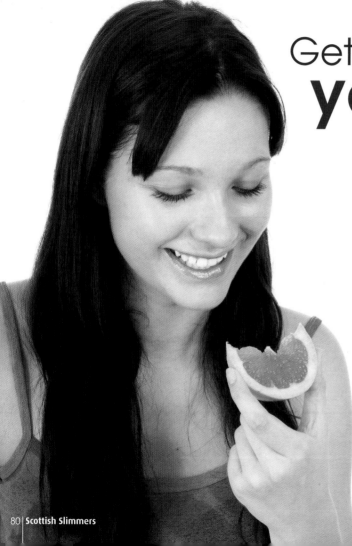

Get the most from
your booster!

Don't forget you also have a Special Weekly Allowance of an extra 20 Checks which can be spent at any time during the week.

Most Essential Extras are counted in exactly the same way as on other Positive Eating Plans, so if you don't want to have those we've included, you can swap these for others with the same Check value.

You don't have to count "No-Need-To-Count" foods, but we recommend you don't have excessively large portions which could slow down your weight loss.

Eggs are a "No-Need-To-Count" food but we recommend that you don't have more than 7 per week.

Every Day Bonus foods should be eaten as usual (they don't have to come out of your daily 20 Checks allowance, or 30 for men).

Every Day Bonus ½ pint skimmed milk, or equivalent in yoghurt/low-fat cheese, is the minimum you should have each day, but as low-fat dairy foods are "No-Need-To-Count" on this Booster Plan, you can have more if you wish!

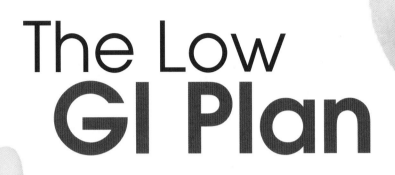

The Low
GI Plan

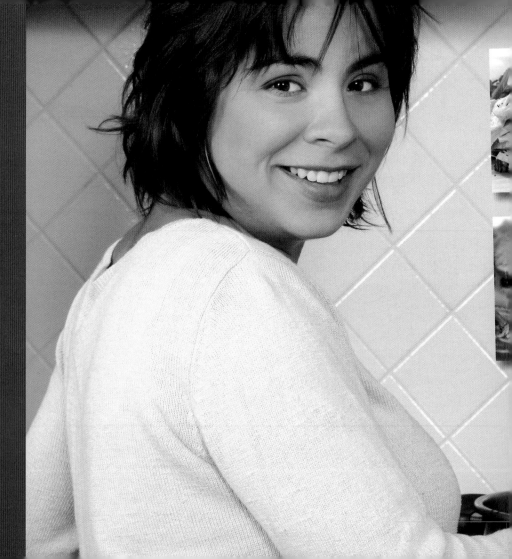

Including lots of low and medium GI (Glycaemic Index) foods in your eating plan can help control cravings, making it easier to lose weight. In this plan, we show you the best foods to choose, most of the time, if you want to go low-GI.

This 7-day example of low-GI eating is based on an average of 40 Checks a day and also includes Every Day Bonus (EDB) foods. Meals may be swapped for others of a similar Check value. Use the GI food lists on page 88 as a guide to making lower GI choices. If you are allowed more Checks than 40, simply choose additional Essential Extras.

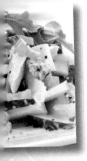
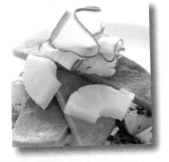

Keeping it **low**

The Glycaemic Index relates only to foods with a high carbohydrate content such as sugar, breads, cereals, flour, pasta, rice, potatoes, fruit and vegetables. Remember, though, that an overall healthy diet does not focus only on one type of nutrient – it's still important to keep down your overall intake of fats, especially saturated animal fats, and to include a wide variety of food.

The way you cook your food and what you eat with it, can also affect the GI rating of a food:

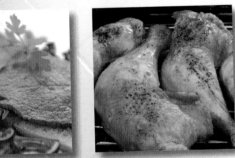

The more you peel and chop carbohydrate foods, and the longer you cook them, the higher their GI rating will be (because there's less work for your digestive system to do).

High fibre foods tend to have a lower GI rating.

Eating some protein (such as meat, fish, pulses, eggs, cheese, milk) with your carbs lowers their overall GI rating. Mixing low GI foods with high GI foods, gives you a medium GI rating.

Acidic foods lower the GI rating – so keep using low-fat vinaigrettes or balsamic vinegar or lemon juice on your salads.

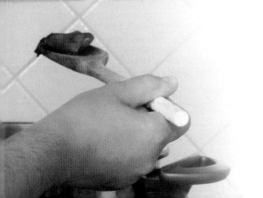

Don't fall into the trap of thinking that you can eat unlimited amounts of low GI carbs – they still have a Check value and, just like any other food, will slow down your weight loss if eaten to excess!

Small between-meal snacks can help keep blood sugars on an even keel. Our plan shows how you can use Every Day Bonus foods to fill the gap.

Eating low GI can help most people but may be especially helpful for those who need to control their blood sugar levels, such as those with metabolic syndrome, insulin resistance, diabetes or PCOS.

MONDAY

EDB **150ml skimmed milk for use in drinks**

8 **3** **Muesli & milk**

45g no-added-sugar muesli with 150ml skimmed milk.

EDB **1 apple**

12 **5** **Chicken tikka pitta**

Cut 1 pitta bread in half to form 2 pockets. Fill with shredded lettuce, cucumber, 100g chicken tikka mini fillets, 2 tsp low-fat natural yoghurt or fromage frais. If you like, add spring onions and a couple of dabs of mint sauce.

EDB **85g grapes**

13 **3** **Haddock with citrus sauce**

Steam or microwave 175g haddock fillet. In a saucepan, mix 1 tsp cornflour and 1/2 tsp stock granules with 125ml unsweetened orange juice. Bring to the boil, stirring continuously, until thickened. Stir in a squeeze of lemon juice and chopped parsley or mint. Serve with 200g new potatoes and green beans or other No-Check vegetables.

EDB **125g pot diet yoghurt**

7 **9** 2 oatcakes with 30g half-fat cheese.

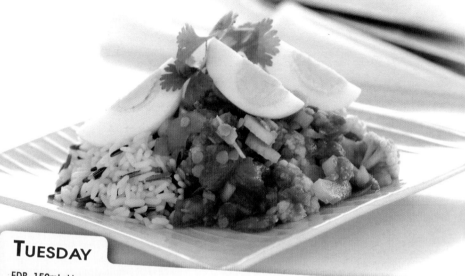

TUESDAY

EDB **150ml skimmed milk for use in drinks**

7 **6** **Cheese on toast**

Melt 30g half-fat cheese on 1 medium slice multigrain or wholemeal toast. Serve with grilled tomatoes.

EDB **1 orange**

11 **11** **Ryvita & pâté**

60g reduced-fat Brussels or Ardennes pâté. Serve with 6 Ryvita Dark Rye crispbreads and No-Check salad.

EDB **1 apple**

16 **14** **Egg & red lentil curry**

Hard boil 1 medium egg. Boil 30g red lentils with 60g each chopped onion, cauliflower and finely sliced celery in 300ml vegetable stock, about 15 minutes. Stir in 200g chopped tomatoes and 1 tsp curry paste. Simmer 10 minutes. Serve with 50g dry weight basmati rice and garnish with quartered egg.

EDB **100g pot diet fromage frais**

5 **5** 2 McVitie's Light Digestives

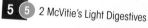

WEDNESDAY

EDB 150ml skimmed milk for use in drinks

8 5 Porridge

Porridge made with 40g oats, water, 150ml skimmed milk, salt or sweetener to taste.

EDB 85g grapes

10 8 Cheese & tomato sandwich

Spread 2 medium slices multigrain or wholemeal bread with 1 tsp low-fat spread and fill with 30g half-fat cheese and tomato slices. Season with black pepper.

EDB 2 small kiwi fruits

16 7 Gammon steak with sweet potato wedges

Boil 200g sweet potato. Drain, cut into wedges, spray lightly with oil and brown under a hot grill. Grill 150g fat-trimmed gammon steak. Serve with 2 tbsp peas and other No-Check vegetables.

EDB 125g pot diet yoghurt

8 14 50g nuts and raisins

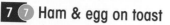

THURSDAY

EDB 150ml skimmed milk for use in drinks

7 7 Ham & egg on toast

Place a thin slice of lean ham on 1 medium slice multigrain or wholemeal toast and top with a poached or microwaved medium egg.

EDB 1 orange

12 10 Sandwich USA

Fill 2 medium slices multigrain or wholemeal bread with 1 dspn peanut butter and 2 tsp jam or fruit spread.

EDB 1 pear

14 7 Steak, fresh tomato & basil pasta

Boil 60g pasta until al dente. Cut 100g lean rump steak into small strips. Heat ½ tsp olive oil and sear steak quickly. Add crushed garlic and 85g fresh chopped tomatoes and cook 2 minutes. Season with salt and black pepper, add 6 large torn basil leaves and cook 1 minute. Serve with drained pasta.

EDB 100g pot diet fromage frais

5 5 2 McVitie's Light Digestives

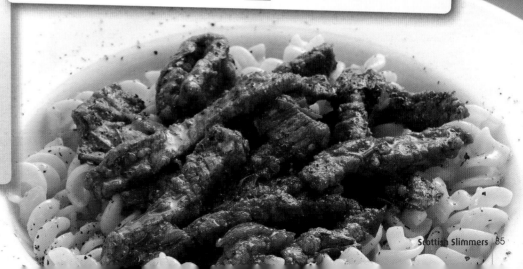

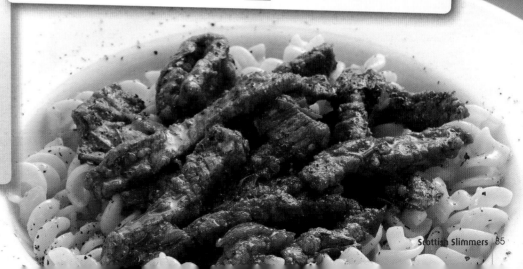

Low GI Plan

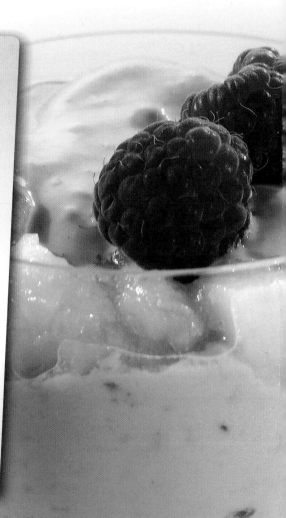

FRIDAY

EDB 150ml skimmed milk for use in drinks

8 8 Oatcakes & soft cheese

3 Paterson's Oatcakes spread with 50g
Philadelphia Extra Light Soft Cheese.

EDB 1 apple

11 12 Houmous & pitta

Serve 1 pitta bread with 2 rounded tbsp
reduced-fat houmous and No-Check salad.

EDB 1 orange

15 9 Red Pesto Chicken

Slit 1 skinless chicken breast horizontally
and fill with 1 dspn red pesto and chopped
mushroom. Wrap 2 turkey rashers around
breast and bake in a moderate oven approx.
25 minutes. Boil and slice 200g new potatoes.
Spray pan with oil and brown potato slices and
slices of courgette.

EDB 125g pot diet yoghurt

5 3 1 medium slice multigrain or
wholemeal toast with 1 tsp low-fat
spread and 1 tsp jam or fruit spread.

SATURDAY

EDB 150ml skimmed milk for use in drinks

8 0 Stewed apple & yoghurt

Stew or microwave 1 cooking apple and serve
topped with 200g pot Mullerlight yoghurt.

EDB 85g grapes

9 1 Pasta & bean soup

Cook together 45g pasta shapes, 3 rounded
tbsp canned kidney beans, 175g chopped
No-Check vegetables, 200g canned tomatoes,
300ml water or stock and pinch herbs. Bring to
the boil then simmer until vegetables and pasta
are cooked.

EDB 100g pot diet fromage frais

**16 16 Pork satay
with basmati rice**

Grill 100g lean pork cubes. Put 1 chopped
spring onion, 1 tbsp peanut butter, 150ml
chicken stock and pinch of chilli into a saucepan. Cook and stir until sauce thickens. Serve
pork with sauce, 35g dry weight boiled basmati
rice and No-Check vegetables.

EDB 2 small kiwi fruits

8 14 50g nuts and raisins

SUNDAY

EDB 150ml skimmed milk for use in drinks

8 3 Breakfast pitta

Spray a pan with oil and cook 1 small sliced onion. Add chopped mushrooms, tomatoes and 2 chopped turkey rashers. Stir-fry a further 2 minutes then serve piled over or in a warmed pitta bread.

EDB 125g pot diet yoghurt

12 12 Salmon & new potato salad

Boil 150g new potatoes. Drain then roughly chop and mix with chopped spring onion and 2 dspn low-calorie mayonnaise. Serve with 75g drained weight canned pink salmon and No-Check salad.

16 10 Souvlaki with couscous & grilled peppers

Marinade 100g cubed lean lamb in 2 tbsp red wine, crushed garlic and good pinch oregano 1 hour or overnight. Thread lamb onto skewers. Cut 1 pepper into eighths. Grill lamb and peppers approx. 15 minutes, turning occasionally. Pour 150ml hot chicken stock over 40g couscous. Cover and leave 10-15 minutes to absorb.

EDB 1 medium banana

 4 2 150g pot low-fat custard

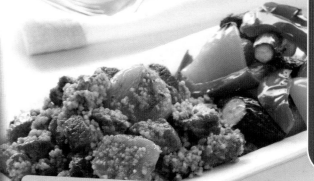

ESSENTIAL EXTRAS

1 slice Burgen Soya & Linseed bread	4	3.5
1 slice Soreen Sliced & Easy	4	0.5
1 pitta bread filled with salad	6	2
1 Laughing Cow Light cheese triangle sandwiched between 2 Ryvita Dark Rye	3	1
2 Paterson's Oatcakes with 15g half-fat cheese	6	6
100-115g mini corn-on-the-cob with 1 tsp low-fat spread	4	3
1 rich tea biscuit	1.5	1.5
1 McVitie's Light Digestive	2.5	2.5
25g nuts & raisins	4	7
25g sunflower or pumpkin seeds	6	12
150g pot low-fat custard	4	2
Sugar-free jelly	No-Check	

GI Food Lists

Low GI

Pumpernickle bread	Apples
Chapatti	Pears
Bran cereals	Apricots
Muesli (no-added-sugar)	Plums
Porridge oats	Berries
Special K	Cherries
Basmati rice	Citrus fruits
Bulghur wheat	Grapes
Noodles	Kiwi fruit
Pasta (al dente)	Mango
Pearl barley	Peaches
Semolina	Nectarines
New potatoes, fresh	Avocados
Sweet potatoes	Olives
Yams	Nuts
Most beans/pulses	Seeds
Lentils	Skimmed milk
Chickpeas	Semi-skimmed milk
Peas	Yoghurt
Sweetcorn	Fromage frais
	Tofu
	Soya Protein
	Digestive biscuits
	Rich tea biscuits
	Fructose

Due to their high water content most vegetables can be treated as low GI

Medium GI

Granary/wholegrain/multigrain bread
Pitta bread
Rye bread
Seeded breads
Tortillas, wraps
Wholemeal bread
Malt loaf
Oatcakes
Ryvita
Weetabix
Shredded Wheat
Brown rice
White & wild rice
Wheat grains
Couscous
Taco shells
New potatoes, canned
Dried fruit
Firm bananas
Pineapple
Yellow/green melons
Honey
Jam/fruit spreads
Plain ice cream
Sugar

High GI

White bread
French bread
Rice cakes
Cornflakes
Puffed wheat
Puffed rice
White rice
Millet
Canned pasta
Jacket baked potatoes
Mashed potatoes
Instant mash
Broad beans
Parsnips
Red/orange melons
Ripe bananas

Zero GI

Lean meat
Poultry
Fish/seafood
Eggs
Low-fat cheeses
Low-fat spreads
Oils

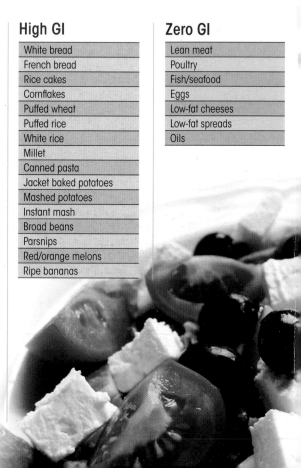